Risk, Age and Pregnancy

Also by Bob Heyman

RESEARCHING USER PERSPECTIVES ON COMMUNITY HEALTH CARE (*editor*)
RISK, HEALTH AND HEALTH CARE: A Qualitative Approach (*editor*)

Risk, Age and Pregnancy

A Case Study of Prenatal Genetic Screening and Testing

Bob Heyman
Professor of Health Research and
Associate Dean for Research
St Bartholomew's School of Nursing and Midwifery
City University
London

and

Mette Henriksen
Registered midwife, and
Research student
University of Northumbria

Consultant Editor: Jo Campling

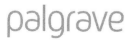

First published 2001 by
PALGRAVE
Houndmills, Basingstoke, Hampshire RG21 6XS and
175 Fifth Avenue, New York, N. Y. 10010
Companies and representatives throughout the world

PALGRAVE is the new global academic imprint of
St. Martin's Press LLC Scholarly and Reference Division and
Palgrave Publishers Ltd (formerly Macmillan Press Ltd).

ISBN 0–333–73940–X

This book is printed on paper suitable for recycling and
made from fully managed and sustained forest sources.

A catalogue record for this book is available
from the British Library.

Library of Congress Cataloging-in-Publication Data
Heyman, Bob.
    Risk, age, and pregnancy : a case study of prenatal genetic
    screening and testing / Bob Heyman, Mette Henriksen.
        p. cm.
    Includes bibliographical references and index.
    ISBN 0–333–73940–X
    1. Genetic screening. 2. Prenatal diagnosis. 3. Pregnancy–
    –Complications. 4. Pregnancy in middle age. I. Henriksen,
    Mette. II. Title.
    RG556 .H49 2000
    618.2'075—dc21
                                                    00–066560

10   9   8   7   6   5   4   3   2   1
10   09 08 07 06 05 04 03 02 01

Printed and bound in Great Britain by
Antony Rowe Ltd, Chippenham, Wiltshire

For Ruth, Michael, Anna, Daniel, Jake, Bent and Hanne

Contents

List of Figures

List of Tables

Acknowledgements

We would like to thank all those who have helped us to write this book: particularly, Susan Fairgrieve and Irene White of the Northern Genetics Service for their generosity with time and advice; Jane Sandall of City University for her constructive comments; and, above all, the pregnant women, doctors and the midwives who shared their views and experiences with us. Responsibility for the content rests solely with the authors.

Introduction

Scope of the book

Aim

Population-based screening systems provide one of the primary means through which risk-oriented societies attempt to organise human services in order to maintain public and individual safety. Such systems scan populations in order to identify sub-populations deemed to face a higher probability of a selected adverse event, and target them for preventative action. A large, rapidly growing research literature (see below) has concerned itself with the formal design and operation of screening systems, for example with rates of take-up, false positives and false negatives. Very little research has explored the organisational complexity of their operation. In consequence, the relationship between screening system blueprints and their manifestation in practice remains unexamined.

The present book will explore this issue through a detailed case study of a genetic screening and testing system for Down's syndrome and other chromosomal abnormalities within one maternity hospital in North-east England. Simple generalisations cannot be drawn from a single case study. But this design does bring the totality of a preventative system into view, and so contributes to a neglected, but theoretically and practically important, issue.

The study focuses on risk management, not the ethical issues surrounding genetic screening for Down's syndrome which have been well discussed elsewhere (for example, Lippman, 1994; Kolker and Burke, 1994; Rothenberg and Thomson, 1994; Bailey, 1996; Malm, 1999). In brief, the present authors support the pro-choice position with respect to abortion, whilst, at the same time, agreeing with the emphasis placed by the social model of disability (Oliver, 1990) on the rights, as against the limitations, of disabled people. We value the potential of the new genetics to reduce human suffering, and fear its eugenic implications. We comfort ourselves with the thought that this subscription to a contradictory set of beliefs is far from unique.

From case to population-based human services

Castel (1991) has identified a phase shift in the relationship between modern health-care systems and their users. During the nineteenth century, professionals saw themselves, primarily, as dealing with individual cases, each characterised by a unique constellation of symptoms, signs, personal qualities and biographical history. Gigerenzer *et al.*, (1990, p. 46) have described the strength of medical opposition, during the first part of the nineteenth century, to the application of the new science of statistics in their field. Doctors of the time believed that statistical approaches could not deal with exceptions, and that the meaning of health could only be defined individually. During the twentieth century, according to Castel, this traditional mode of relating has become transformed into one in which professionals, guided by epidemiological analysis of risk factors, screen, select from and process populations. As a result, he argues, the individual has disappeared from the view of service providers, and has become merely the intersection of a set of risk factors within processed populations. Although Castel's analysis was developed in the context of mental health services, it applies at least as well to medicine based on the new genetics. As one expert quoted by Ettore (1999, p. 549) put it:

> *Screening is an opportunity for preventing a serious disease . . . My approach* [to prenatal genetic screening] *is basically as a mass medical activity . . . This is still very much a specialist area covered by the clinical genetics discipline.*

Remarkably, one of our respondents, a pregnant midwife, identified just this transition, which she saw as a means of managing scarce caring resources more efficiently, and, thus, as an adaptation to the demands of mass health care.

Pregnant midwife: *We've gone to, sort of, seeing pregnancy as a risk, and bring them back to the clinic every few weeks, and where most of the care is mostly done in the community. And these women* [seen in the community] *are classed as low risk pregnancies. And we are seeing now, I would say, more and more of the higher risk pregnancies, rather than the low risk pregnancies, which is good really, because you don't have those horrendous clinics like we used to have . . . You could be here four or five hours.* (Shirley, midwife, aged 34, interview, 20 weeks, no genetic tests)

The extent of the demise of the individual from the view of health and social care professionals should not be exaggerated. Our own findings (see Chapter 3) suggest that, in current maternity services at least, idiographic, case-based and nomothetic, population-based approaches to care for pregnant women and their babies may coexist, although often uneasily, and sometimes with bizarre consequences, such as the use of screening as a medical response to general anxiety. Nevertheless, an enormous expansion in the range of screening programmes is currently taking place. A historical excavation in the Medline database, the results of which are summarised in Figure 0.1, illustrates this trend.

The above graph compares the rate of change in the number of outputs discussing human screening systems and neoplasms during the 1980s and 90s. The latter is included as a control indicative of the general trend of change in the number of reported outputs concerned with curative medical treatment. As can be seen, recorded neoplasm

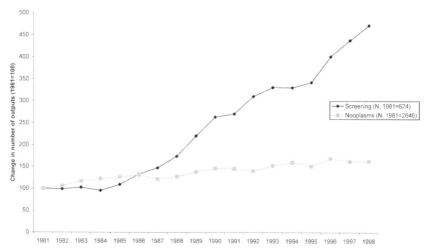

Figure 0.1 Change in number of screening and neoplasm outputs from the Medline database 1981–98

research output increased steadily, by over 50 per cent, whilst the level of screening research output started to accelerate in 1984, generating nearly a 500 per cent increase during this period. The graph documents the impact of the risk society (Beck, 1992) on the organisation of health care.

The shift towards screening populations identified by Castel (1991) can be observed in many spheres of health and social care. For example, a search of the Medline database using the keyword *'screening'*, listed on one page studies of: low birth weight (Lawoyin, 1998); coronary heart disease (Lee *et al.*, 1999); breast cancer (Decker, Harrison and Tate, 1999); neonatal hearing disorders (Meyer *et al.*, 1999); domestic violence (Siegel *et al.*, 1999); and prostate cancer (Anonymous, 1999).

Comparisons of different types of screening system can be expected to reveal common characteristics, such as tension between providers of systems which are oriented to populations and service users who insist on regarding themselves as cases, as already mentioned. At the same time, the character of a screening system will be affected by the nature of the risk it is designed to minimise. Screening systems for infectious diseases, mental health problems and genetic abnormalities, for example, give rise to quite different policy, organisational, communication and ethical issues.

The Geneticisation of Pregnancy

The present case study is concerned with the management of genetic risks which cannot be treated. It, therefore, has implications for the class of screening systems based on the new genetics (Lenaghan, 1998), a class which, for better or worse, can be expected to expand rapidly during the first decades of the new millennium. Inevitably, the advent of new genetic technologies will strengthen the trend towards geneticisation (Lippman, 1994), the tendency to view all human problems through a genetic prism. This trend will, in turn, stimulate sharp questioning of the relationship between medical innovation and medical progress.

The characteristics of screening systems designed to reduce the risk of babies being born with serious chromosomal abnormalities such as trisomy 21 will be explored in some detail in the pages that follow. At this point, we will do no more than briefly raise two major strategic issues associated with the development and operation of such systems.

Firstly, prenatal genetic screening systems, although now routine in maternity care within most, but not all, Western societies, provide a radically new, but highly imperfect, form of control over the human condition. Limited knowledge about the genetic makeup of a baby can be obtained before it is born. But this knowledge is used mainly to terminate affected pregnancies, not to treat genetic conditions. Because no treatment of choice can be offered, parents are faced with the dilemma of declining genetic tests, accepting the risk that a baby with chromosomal abnormalities will be born, as against going down a road which might begin with genetic screening, but which could end up with abortion. Beck-Gernsheim (1996), drawing on the work of Beck (1992), sees this historically novel burden of decision-making now placed on parents as an example of individualisation, a wider societal process in which individuals and families are required to take responsibility for managing an ever-increasing range of contingencies.

Prenatal genetic testing makes parents responsible for their children's chromosomes. Our case study will document the ways in which they cope with this shift within a specific screening system context. However, responsibility is not shared equally. In theory, pregnant women may take, or have no choice but to take, this burden onto themselves, may share responsibility with their partner, or may find that he takes responsibility away from them. Although all three patterns will be documented in our case study, the first appears to predominate. Responsibility for genetic decision-making, as with other positively or negatively valued social roles, is not distributed equally.

A second characteristic marking out the type of screening under investigation is the pace of technical and organisational change in the field. The hospital site for our research offered prenatal serum screening and amniocentesis (see below) routinely to women aged 35 and over in the second trimester of their pregnancy. Since the time when the main fieldwork for the present study was undertaken, in 1995–97, the routine offering of serum screening to women of all ages has become more common; as have first semester serum screening and the measurement of nuchal translucency via scans (Spencer *et al.*, 1999; Wald, 1999).

Despite the radical novelty of prenatal genetic screening and testing within the wider society, our study offers a social history of the use of a disappearing technology (although the screening system at our hospital research site remained, in the year 2000, essentially the same as the one we analysed). Indeed, social scientists, like those who organise screening systems, are faced with a pace of change which renders their efforts old-fashioned just as they are bearing fruit. Our defence of the value of the present work is not that it illuminates the workings of a particular system but that it can shed light on the operation of any probabilistic screening system designed to prevent infrequent events.

No generalisations can be made from the study about the current state of prenatal screening and testing in the UK or elsewhere. However, we hope that it will cast a little light, more generally, on the nature of systems designed to screen populations in order to reduce risk.

Scope of the Introduction

The rest of this introductory chapter will: firstly, discuss the terminological problems which bedevil genetic discourse; secondly, introduce a theoretical framework which treats risk as a social resource rather than a natural phenomenon; thirdly, summarise the methodology of the case study around which the book is written; and, fourthly, outline the structure of the book.

Terminological politics

Investigators of the operation of health and social care systems invariably find themselves travelling through terminological minefields, particularly when contentious issues such as disability and abortion are involved (Heyman, 1995). The main choices which anyone discussing prenatal screening/testing for Down's syndrome must make are summarised in Table 0.1, and briefly discussed below.

The word *'foetus'* refers to a biological organism, whereas a *'baby'* possesses personhood and human rights. These terms do not merely describe but carry with them attitudes to the entity referenced. People in Western cultures do not describe a birth at term as happening to a foetus, and only a minority think of a newly fertilised human egg as a baby. For most, a mysterious transformation from foetus to baby takes place at some time in the pregnancy, not necessarily at the legal limit,

Table 0.1   Terminological options in the language of screening/testing for Down's syndrome

Foetus	Baby
Pregnancy termination	Abortion
Trisomy 21	Down's syndrome
Handicap	Disability
Risk	Probability
Screening	Testing
Higher/lower risk	Positive/negative test result
Hospital consultation	Genetic counselling
Older mother	Mature mother
Patient	Pregnant woman

24 weeks in the UK unless the foetus has an abnormality (HMSO, 1990). One health professional with whom we discussed our research findings insisted that a foetus should only be described as a baby, and its progenitors as parents, after pregnancy termination had been ruled out. Similarly, some of our respondents (see Chapter 5) held back from identifying with their baby until they had received genetic test results, thus maintaining the status of their progeny as a foetus until this time. Others felt emotionally attached to their baby from the start of their pregnancy. Hence, the status of foetus/baby cannot be linked to its inherent characteristics, but to the alternative way in which parents and others think about this entity.

The terms *'pregnancy termination'* and *'abortion'* in Table 0.1 apply to foetuses and babies respectively, conveying the switching off of a biological process and the destruction of a life respectively. Trisomy 21 refers to the genetic cause of Down's syndrome, and the latter term to its highly variable consequences. The former draws attention to genetic processes and the latter to their bio-social meaning. Our respondents, both pregnant women and doctors, sometimes used the term 'handi-capped' to describe a person with Down's syndrome, despite the efforts of the WHO to differentiate handicap from disability (WHO, 1980). This epithet conveys a belief that functional deficits arise directly from a medical condition. It therefore discounts the influence of societal processes which may counteract or reinforce the effects of disability caused by biological impairment.

The next two couplets in Table 0.1 appertain to the preventative system for Down's syndrome. 'Probability' refers, with apparent neu-trality, to the likelihood that a future or otherwise unknown event will take place. (We will question this neutrality below.) Risks, in contrast, may be acceptable if weighed against the costs of prevention, but, *ceteris paribus*, should be avoided. The depiction of the probability of Down's syndrome as a risk, thus smuggles in an unexamined negative value judgement about the adversity of the condition.

A distinction, by no means clear-cut, can be drawn between screen-ing a population for a condition and testing individuals who are sus-pected of having it (Lenaghan, 1998, p. 24). A screening system may be accepted despite having limited accuracy because it allows a sub-population at higher risk of a condition to be targeted from more inva-sive, but also more accurate, diagnostic tests which deliver a definitive verdict. As the hospital doctors who advised the pregnant women in our study often pointed out, a 'higher risk' serum screening outcome must be distinguished from a 'positive' amniocentesis diagnosis. Most women placed into the higher risk serum screening category will not give birth to a baby with Down's syndrome (see next section). This screening outcome should not, strictly speaking, be described as a false positive. Similarly, some 'lower risk' women will, by definition, give birth to babies with Down's syndrome, an outcome which cannot be accurately described as a 'false negative'.

Doctors at our hospital research site, however, did refer to false positive and negative serum screening test results, as does the medical literature (Wald and Hackshaw, 1997). Questions about the legitimacy of the current serum screening system underlie this terminological confusion. Distress during the waiting period of up to three weeks between receiving a higher risk screening result and obtaining a definitive diagnosis of amniocentesis may be reduced, or at least de-emphasised, if women are told that they are at higher risk rather than that they have tested positive. Green (1994) found that 80 per cent of obstetric consultants felt that pregnant women would not fully understand the probabilistic logic which underlies serum screening. In particular, they believed that women may suffer unnecessary anxiety because they treat a 'higher risk' screening as equivalent to a 'positive' test result. Some researchers have reported that women find this outcome highly distressing (Abuelo *et al.*, 1991; Marteau *et al.*, 1992a; Statham and Green, 1993; Santalahti *et al.*, 1996), although one recent study concluded that only 3 per cent of women who screen positive suffer a serious psychological reaction (Goel *et al.*, 1998). The extent to which any distress experienced can be reduced by presentational means is questionable.

To complicate terminological matters still further, an accurate test such as amniocentesis can be used to screen a population as well as to diagnose the presence of a condition in individuals classified as being at higher risk. Moreover, the main current screening technique is commonly referred to as a blood test. In an attempt to combine economy with clarity, we will mostly refer to the combined system of probabilistic screening and diagnostic testing for chromosomal abnormalities as 'genetic screening/testing' and to the procedures used as 'genetic tests'.

The next terminological choice listed in Table 0.1 concerns the description of the advice which women receive, at our hospital research site, from hospital doctors, as 'counselling'. The Northern Genetics Service (personal communication, 1999) advised us not to describe these discussions as genetic counselling, but as screening counselling, on the grounds that the former has a wider scope, encompassing problems with specific genes as well as chromosomal abnormalities. They agreed, however, that these encounters, whether involving a midwife or doctor, provided information rather than counselling. We will refer to those provided at our research site as hospital consultations, and never as counselling.

Our next terminological minefield references the highly sensitive issue of the marking out of some pregnant women on account of their age. Political correctness would, today, make obviously unacceptable the decision made by the International Council of Obstetricians and Gynaecologists in 1958, that a woman aged 35 years or older at her first delivery was to be called an *'elderly primigravida'*, and considered a high risk patient (Tuck, Yudkin and Turnbull, 1988). Nevertheless, many women do feel stigmatised on account of their age, as will be seen in Chapter 2. Some point out the positive advantages of being older, such as greater experience and maturity. Hence, a woman might be defined as, or see herself as being, 'older', a term which we gloss as a modern euphemism for 'elderly'. The alternative term, 'mature', conveys a positive stance towards this chronology. Whatever terms are used, the division of pregnant women into age groups requires the setting of arbitrary and debatable dividing lines which cut up and homogenise the continuous flow of time.

Finally, women having babies in hospital are sometimes called 'patients', with the implication that they are suffering from a health problem requiring medical intervention. Use of terms such as 'patient', 'client', 'consumer', 'customer' and even 'punter' conveys differing implicit assumptions about relationships between them and service providers (Heyman, 1995, p. 18). Throughout the book, we will refer to those attending hospital in order to have a baby as 'pregnant women'.

Language packages together description and evaluation, causing problems for social scientists who wish to explore value differences. We will employ terms such as 'baby' and 'foetus', 'higher risk' and 'screen positive' interchangeably, in the hope that the reader will bear in mind the health warning on language usage which we have provided.

Down's syndrome and genetic screening/testing

In this section, we will, firstly, discuss the broader context of pregnancy screening and testing; secondly, briefly consider present medical knowledge about the nature of Down's syndrome; and, finally, outline the main features of the genetic screening/testing system for this condition at our hospital research site.

Pregnancy risk management

From a current obstetric perspective, pregnancy may be viewed primarily as a process which generates risks for the mother and baby (Tew, 1990, p. 11). Risk reduction strategies in modern maternity hospitals often entail the organisation of procedures for detecting and preventing medical problems in the population of pregnant women and babies. Inevitably, risks are selectively focused upon in such systems, with the degree of attention affected by technical, economic, organisational and cultural factors. Thus, for very different reasons, cystic fibrosis and postnatal depression are, at the time of writing, not generally screened for in the population of UK pregnant women, despite the availability of tests, and the very high prevalence of the latter condition, which affects 35 per cent of women according to one Australian survey (Horan-Smith and Gullone, 1998).

Populations, or large sub-populations, of pregnant women in most Western societies are offered a wide range of screening tests, for conditions detected primarily by scan, for example, spina bifida; for chromosomal abnormalities diagnosed through chorionic villus sampling or amniocentesis, for example Down's and Edward's syndrome; and for infectious diseases, most recently HIV. Pregnant women provide the most fully developed exemplar of an intersection of risk factors (Castel, 1991). The prevailing neo-liberalism, on which the current organisation of health and social care is predicated, treats the individual as a rational, autonomous decision-maker (Petersen, 1999) whose choices are based on an understanding of his or her rights and obligations as a citizen, and the digestion of packaged but objective scientific information. This world view treats rationality as solely calculative, rather than as built on a bedrock of socially mediated prior assumptions.

The impact of the 'new genetics', fuelled by the mapping of the human genome, can only increase the range of foetal conditions which are screened for, making it more difficult to draw the dividing line between acceptable and unacceptable genetic variations (Marteau and Richards, 1996). This development raises questions about who defines 'good' and 'bad' genes, and to what ends (Willis, 1998). Lippman (1994, p. 144) coined the phrase '*geneticization*' to describe a mind-set in which '*differences between individuals are reduced to their DNA codes, with most disorders, behaviours and physiological variations defined, at least in part, as genetic in origin*'. Genetic explanations support the individualistic cultural perspective, prevalent in the USA and, to a lesser extent, the

UK, which explains social problems in terms of attributes of individuals (Nelkin and Lindee, 1998, p. 194).

The most widely used application of genetic technology is, at the present time, in prenatal diagnosis. The concept of geneticisation can be further developed from a risk perspective. It will be argued, in Chapter 1, that women will have their attention selectively drawn to those risks which available genetic technology is applied to. Hence, for example, women will be asked to worry about Down's syndrome, but not about cystic fibrosis, for which population screening, although available, is not currently provided in most areas of the UK. By implication, as the scope and availability of genetic screening/testing technologies expands, parents will be expected to concern themselves about the prevention of more and more conditions. This expansion of responsibility for what might previously have been regarded as random contingencies belongs to a wider shift towards screening for risk factors, as already noted.

The geneticisation of childbirth can be criticised on three grounds. Firstly, it directs attention selectively to the prevention of genetic risks, whilst other risks to the health and welfare of the child, for example those arising from maternal poverty, are ignored (Lippman, 1994). Secondly, it places parents under intense pressure, requiring them to take individual responsibility for managing an ever-widening range of genetic risks (Beck-Gernsheim, 1996). Thirdly, genetic screening and testing is predicated on eugenic values which legitimate the view that certain categories of people may beneficially be eliminated from the population. As the scope of genetic screening/testing expands, more and more people become '*abortable*' (Black, 1979), and '*the notion that genetic counsellors can, and should be, value-free and non-directive will become more and more difficult to sustain*' (Petersen, 1999, p. 263). Damage may be done to all those people who are missed by the filter of prevention, and who arrive in a world which has developed procedures to prevent their existence (Rothman, 1988). (Defenders of genetic screening/testing can argue, however, that societies can afford to provide better support for a reduced population of people with medical and functional problems.) Thirdly, genes can only be expressed in an environment. Judgements about the abortability of those with a particular genetic condition inadvertently incorporate the influence of current social conditions, and the limitations they impose upon human potential, itself an unknowable and theoretically unlimited quality (Heyman, Huckle and Handyside, 1998). For example, people with Down's syndrome living in Western societies currently enjoy a greatly extended life expectancy, due to medical advances, but suffer isolation from the economic mainstream which results in limited life opportunities.

Down's syndrome

Down's syndrome is only one of a wide range of chromosomal abnormalities which, overall, affect 6 out of every 1000 births (Tolmie, 1995). Hence, the concentration of attention on this risk (see *'Selective Attention to Down's Syndrome'* in Chapter 1) entails a double act of choice, firstly of genetic conditions, and, secondly, of one particular chromosomal problem. We will argue, in Chapter 1, that this doubly selective risk attention is driven by the availability of screening/testing systems. The risk status of Down's syndrome is, thus, generated by the efforts made to prevent it.

The incidence of Down's syndrome births

Down's syndrome is caused by a reproductive malfunction in which the fertilised egg contains three copies of the 21st chromosome instead of the usual two. Because the extra chromosome is donated most commonly by the mother, the incidence of Down's syndrome is related more closely to maternal than to paternal age. A small but substantial over-representation of male compared with female births, of the order of about 1.2 to 1 has been found (Robinson, 1996). In the absence of selective abortion, a rate of 1.4 per 1000 live births can be expected, generating about 1000 babies with Down's syndrome per year in the UK (Cuckle, 1997). However, this rate depends upon the profile of risk factors in the population of pregnant women, particularly the maternal age distribution (Cuckle, Wald and Thompson, 1987). Currently, the reduction in the rate of births of babies with Down's syndrome resulting from screening/testing a higher proportion of the population is counterbalanced by the trend towards later child-birth.

To complicate matters further, the pre-test probability that a woman is carrying a baby with Down's syndrome changes during the course of the pregnancy. This change arises from the relatively high probability that foetuses with genetic abnormalities will be aborted spontaneously. Studies of pregnancy outcomes among women who did not abort after Down's syndrome was diagnosed through amniocentesis or chorionic villus sampling, together with cross-sectional comparisons at different pregnancy stages, allow survival chances to be estimated. About 40 per cent of Down's syndrome babies identified at 10 weeks' gestation, and 20 per cent of those detected at 16 weeks, are aborted spontaneously or stillborn (Noble, 1998). As a result, the probability of a still pregnant woman giving birth to a baby with Down's syndrome increases as she progresses towards term.

Predicting Down's syndrome

Maternal age provides the best predictor of the incidence of Down's syndrome births, but estimates of the probabilities associated with specific ages are surrounded with some uncertainty. The risk statistics developed by Cuckle, Wald and Thompson (1987) were recommended by the Northern Region Genetics Service (1995), and were cited by doctors during hospital consultations. However, estimation of rates for women of specific ages entails a number of methodological complexities, for example, induction from regression equations derived from observation of outcomes in relatively small numbers of pregnant women of specific ages. Alternative maternal age-related probabilities have been proposed (Halliday *et al.*, 1995; Hook and Chambers, 1997).

The causal processes linking maternal age to Down's syndrome are not well understood. Most women, except at the most advanced ages possible, do not give birth to babies with Down's syndrome. In theory, the relationship between maternal age and the condition might not result from intrinsic features of the former. We will illustrate this possibility by outlining the theory of preovulatory overripeness of the human egg (Jongbloet and Zwets, 1976).

According to this theory, a wide range of health problems, including Down's syndrome, become more likely if egg fertilisation takes place towards the end of a woman's menstrual cycle. The average time between release of the egg and conception may increase in the premenopausal period because lengthy menstrual cycles occur more frequently, and/or because coitus occurs less frequently. The preovulatory overripeness theory implies that the association between maternal age and foetal Down's syndrome is merely correlational, arising because older women conceive, on average, later in the menstrual cycle.

If validated, this theory would generate a completely new preventative system, based on the timing of conception in the monthly cycle, rather than on maternal age. We do not seek to advocate the theory, but to illustrate the relevance to risk analysis of the well-known distinction between correlation and causation. Probabilistic prediction requires only correlation. As long as those who are trying to manage the future rest happy with their prognostic power, alternative predictive schema will not be explored. These alternatives can be easily overlooked if the predictors cannot be readily assessed, and/or they do not fit with prevailing research paradigms. Both of these conditions hold with respect to preovulatory overripeness. It requires estimation of the timing of conception in the monthly cycle. And it invokes a medically un-fashionable behavioural explanation (a reduced rate of coitus among older couples) of a chromosomal abnormality.

The incidence of Down's syndrome births is associated with a number of other factors over and above maternal age. These include paternal age (Jalbert, 1996), family history (Cuckle and Wald, 1990), a history of maternal exposure to abdominal X-rays (Rose, 1994) and low-level environmental radiation (Bound, Francis and Harvey, 1995), and conception in the winter months (Puri and Singh, 1995). These variables could, in theory, be included in, and would therefore change, the estimation of Down's syndrome probabilities for individual women. The apparently bizarre idea that the probability of an individual expe-riencing a given event depends upon the information which is consid-ered will be justified below, in the section on *'Risk Knowledge'*, and related to research data in Chapter 4, in the section on *'The Probability Heuristic'*.

The meaning of Down's syndrome

People with Down's syndrome experience varying degrees of intellec-tual disability. Nomothetic comparisons of populations with and without the condition suggest that they are more likely than the general population to encounter a wide range of health problems, including, for example, congenital heart disease (Marino, 1993), leukaemia (Mili, *et al.*, 1993), immune system deficiencies (Nespoli, *et al.*, 1993) and pre-mature ageing (Collacott, Cooper and Ismail, 1994).

However, the biological impact of trisomy 21 varies considerably in individual cases. (The implications of such differences for risk rea-soning will be considered in Chapter 1.) Little is known about the processes linking various types and degrees of chromosome 21 overdose to the occurrence of intellectual and health problems. Studies of rare cases of partial trisomy 21 have been used to specify associations between small regions of chromosome 21 and particular consequences such as intellectual disability and heart problems (Delabar *et al.*, 1993). However, recent research (Greber-Platzer *et al.*, 1999) has not supported the hypothesis of a relationship between gene dosage in a previously identified region and congenital heart disease. Shapiro (1997) noted that no association between an overdose of a specific gene and a feature of the condition has been discovered, and that no health problem other than, possibly, intellectual disability is found in all people with Down's syndrome. He speculated that problems might result simply from the total amount of extra gene transcription caused by the activity, itself variable, of the additional chromosome. We will carry forward the conclusions that probabilistic predictions about the birth of children with Down's syndrome refer to a highly variable phenomenon, and that the underlying causes of this variation are unknown.

The prenatal genetic screening/testing system

The presence of Down's syndrome and other chromosomal conditions in the foetus is, currently, investigated through screening procedures which only estimate the probability of these abnormalities; or through very accurate diagnostic tests, amniocentesis and chorionic villus sampling, which may cause miscarriages. In this section, we will briefly discuss the first two options, largely ignoring chorionic villus sampling, which was only rarely offered at our hospital research site, via another local hospital. We will then consider national and local variation in the specification of genetic screening/testing systems.

Some form of screening/testing for chromosomal abnormalities is offered routinely to some or all pregnant women attending British maternity hospitals. Current practice varies considerably. For example, some hospitals give the option of serum screening to all women, whilst others do not provide it for any women, offering only amniocentesis to women aged 35 and over. Serum screening was offered selectively, at our hospital research site, at around 16 weeks' gestation. Results took about a week to process. Women who screen positive are offered amniocentesis. They must wait up to a further three weeks to learn the outcome of this definitive diagnostic test. Women attending this hospital may also undergo amniocentesis, usually at around 14–18 weeks' gestation, directly, without prior serum screening. This option is more likely to be recommended, and taken up, by women in their late thirties and over, as will be shown in Chapter 4 (see Table 4.1).

Nationally, the proportion of pregnant women offered prenatal screening/testing has gradually increased since the late 1980s. As a result, the percentage of detected cases of Down's syndrome diagnosed prenatally in England and Wales increased from 30 per cent to 53 per cent between 1989 and 1997; and from 9 per cent to 45 per cent between 1987 and 1997 for mothers aged under 35 (Mutton, Ide and Alberman, 1998).

Serum screening methods and amniocentesis, the two main options available at our hospital research site, are discussed briefly below.

Serum screening

The history of maternal serum screening for Down's syndrome has been well summarised by Wald *et al.* (1998). Raised maternal serum levels of alpha-fetoprotein (AFP) were statistically associated with an increased foetal prevalence of neural tube defects and spina bifida during the 1970s, giving rise to screening programmes for these conditions. During the 1980s, it was found that reduced maternal serum levels of this marker were linked to an increased foetal prevalence of trisomy 18, which causes Edward's syndrome, and of the more common trisomy 21, which causes Down's syndrome. Screening programmes began to be implemented in the late 1980s. More markers were soon added to the risk assessment, including maternal serum chorionic gonadotropin (hCG) and unconjugated oestriol (uE_3). Their use in various combinations, together with maternal age, improves screening accuracy. Risk estimation will depend upon which serum markers, for example whole hCG or its breakdown products, a laboratory measures (Spencer, 1997; Wald *et al.*, 1998), and upon measurement factors, discussed below.

Probabilistic inference from serum markers

Because of their imperfect accuracy, screening results relate to the presence of Down's syndrome only probabilistically. A false screen positive arises if a woman who screens positive turns out to be carrying a baby without the chromosomal conditions being tested for, and a false screen negative if a baby with one of these conditions is not identified by the screening process. As noted above, these outcomes should more accurately, but verbosely, be described in terms of probability. For example a screening false positive should be referred to as the placement in the higher risk group of a mother who is not bearing a baby with Down's syndrome.

The interpretation of probabilistic predictions involves complex reasoning which even academic psychologists get wrong (Falk and Greenbaum, 1995; Dracup, 1995). Four types of predictive error are summarised and quantified with respect to serum screening in Table 0.2. The statistics come from a large meta-analysis involving a total of nearly 300 000 women (Cuckle, 1996).

The bifurcation of positive and negative errors shown in the two rows of Table 0.2 is required to take into account two alternative ways of grounding a probability calculation. The probability of A, given B, cannot be equated with the probability of B, given A, although these two para-

Table 0.2   The risk of detection and non-detection errors from serum screening for Down's syndrome

	Detection errors	**Non-detection errors**
Down's syndrome the denominator	The probability that a woman will screen positive even though she does not give birth to a baby with Down's syndrome.	The probability that a woman will screen negative even though she does give birth to a baby with Down's syndrome.
	4.5% (Selectivity = 95.5%)	34% (Sensitivity = 66%)
Test result the denominator	The probability that a woman will not give birth to a baby with Down's syndrome, even though she screened positive.	The probability that a woman will give birth to a baby with Down's syndrome, even though she screened negative.
	98% (Positive predictive value = 2%)	0.05% (Negative predictive value = 99.95%)

meters are often confused (Dracup, 1995). For example, if 1 : 700 women in a screened population gave birth to babies with Down's syndrome, and 4.5 per cent were classified as at higher risk, then, on average, about 32 women out of 700 (4.5 per cent) would falsely screen positive. One of these 700 women would, in the absence of selective abortion, give birth to a baby with Down's syndrome. Therefore, 95 per cent (32 out of 33) women who screened positive would be expected not to give birth to a baby with Down's syndrome. (The slight discrepancies from Table 0.2 occur because these probabilities depend upon the estimated overall Down's syndrome rate.) Moreover, as screening detects only two-thirds of Down's syndrome foetuses, it follows that about 48 women (32/0.66) will falsely screen positive, on average, for every one for whom screening detects correctly. Similarly, a 34 per cent probability of a negative screening result, given the birth of a baby with Down's syndrome, would result in one such birth for every 2100 pregnancies (1 : 700 × 0.34). The overall probability of a Down's syndrome birth given a negative screening result would, therefore, be about 0.05 per cent.

The existence of two types of probability of detection and non-detection error offers a choice of presentation which can be used, consciously or unconsciously, for micro-political purposes, as will be seen in Chapter 7. Research papers extolling the virtues of screening systems for low frequency conditions usually discuss the relatively low rate of false positives, that is, the low proportion of people without the condition who screen positive (high test selectivity). In contrast, mention is rarely given to the much higher proportion of individuals who do not have the condition even though they have screened positive (low positive predictive value). Similarly (see Chapter 7), women who are told that one-third of Down's syndrome cases are not detected through serum screening (that the test has moderate sensitivity) might feel less inclined towards amniocentesis if they realised that, on average, only 1:2000 women who screen negative give birth to a baby with the condition (that the test has very high negative predictive value).

Figure 0.2, based loosely on that displayed by Wald and Hackshaw (1997, p. 46), nicely illustrates how value judgements can be smuggled into apparently descriptive graphical representations of probability distributions.

The differentiation of false positives and negatives is based on a selected probability level, in this case, 1:200. A decision by the architects of the screening system to modify this critical probability would, of course, lead to reclassification of some women between the two risk categories, and would change the overall selectivity and sensitivity of the test.

The distributions shown in Figure 0.2 have been scaled so that their total frequencies, that is, the areas under the curves, appear equal.

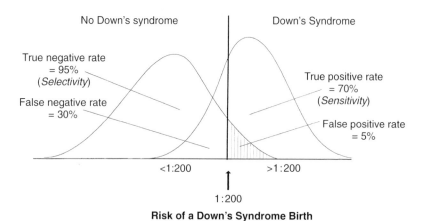

Figure 0.2 A graphical representation of Down's syndrome risk after serum screening

However, only about 1:700 of the current population of pregnant women give birth to a baby with Down's syndrome in the absence of selective abortion. This difference in scale could be represented by making the distribution of unaffected pregnancies 700 times larger than the Down's syndrome distribution! The area corresponding to the false positive rate for unaffected pregnancies would overwhelm the entire latter distribution.

We do not suggest that either probabilistic picture possesses more absolute validity than the other, only that representations of probabilities, including apparently objective, scientific graphs, contain embedded assumptions.

Complications

The probabilistic position discussed above needs to be complicated in two ways. Firstly, the false positive rate increases and the false negative rate decreases with maternal age. For example, in the Northern region of England (Northern Genetics Service, 1998) the false screen positive rate in 1997 ranged from 3 per cent among women aged under 35 to 25 per cent among those aged 38 and over. Age-related false screen negative rate cannot be accurately estimated for the region because of the very low number of cases of the condition (12 in 1997). Our hospital screens selectively, targeting mainly older women (see below), whilst others, both regionally and nationally, offer screening to all women. In consequence, the average age of those screened, and therefore the overall false positive rate, about 9 per cent, was higher than that obtained for the region as a whole, around 5 per cent (Northern Genetics Service, 1998).

Secondly, measurement problems, rarely discussed with pregnant women, affect the estimates of personal probabilities. Problems arise in the assessment of gestational age, which has to be taken into account because of its association with average, expected serum marker levels, and of the serum markers themselves. A crucial factor affecting the accuracy of measurement of gestational age is the use of dating scans. One major regional hospital in NE England did not, at the time of the research, use dating scans to assess foetal age. As a result, it generated a false positive rate almost double that which would have been expected on the basis of the age profile of the women it screened. The false positive rate at our hospital research site closely matched its expected rate (Northern Genetics Service, 1998).

Those who possess little or no biomedical knowledge, including the present authors and most pregnant women, tend to take for granted the accuracy of laboratory measurements. However, quality checks suggest that their reliability can be questioned. Seth and Ellis (1994) compared UK laboratory assessments of parts of the same serum sample. They concluded that the level of agreement was inversely related to the number of serum markers taken into account, being highest for AFP alone, and lowest for the triple combination of AFP, intact hCG and uE_3. They explain this finding by arguing that the increase in the number of analytical steps associated with use of more markers increases the scope for significant procedural variation. This finding raises the disturbing possibility that the use of additional markers to improve predictive accuracy also increases the chance of error. Seth and Ellis (1994) note that resulting differences in pro-bability estimates can significantly affect the classification of marginal cases as at higher or lower risk. For example, the probability of Down's syndrome estimated by different laboratories from one sample through the combination of AFP and intact hCG ranged from $1:115$ to $1:550$. Moreover, errors in measuring serum markers and gesta-tional age will compound each other. These significant measurement problems were not discussed with pregnant women at our hospital research site, and receive little prominence in the literature. The Northern Genetics Service stated (personal communication, 1999) that no consultant had requested copies of Laboratory Performance Reports on the accuracy of serum screening which the Service had offered to provide.

Technical advances

Various ultrasound markers, particularly increased nuchal fold thick-ness, are also coming into use in prenatal genetic screening (Macintosh, 1997). Wald, Watt and Hackshaw (1999) have recently recommended use of a double screening procedure, with nuchal translucency and pregnancy-associated plasma protein A assessed in the first trimester, and the markers mentioned above in the second. They concluded that use of this combination would reduce the proportion of false positives from about 5 per cent to 1 per cent, and the detection rate from 69 per cent to 85 per cent. However, the increase in accuracy resulting from this system, which would reduce the need for invasive diagnostic tests, could be achieved only at the price, for women, of greatly extending the waiting period for screening results, presently one week, to about five weeks.

Spencer *et al.* (1999) have developed a One Stop Counselling, Assess-ment and Risk (OSCAR) system, with risk assessment based on the plasma protein-A combination of first trimester maternal serum screening, maternal age and foetal nuchal translucency. A different set of serum markers (free betahuman chorionic gonadotropin and pregnancy-associated plasma protein-A) from those measured in second trimester screening is assessed automatically, allowing results to be returned within 30 minutes. Spencer *et al.* report improved accuracy from this system compared with one based on maternal second semester serum screening and age. OSCAR allows a 1 per cent false positive rate to be achieved with a detection rate of 70 per cent, or a 5 per cent false positive rate to be traded against a detection rate of 90 per cent, depending upon where the boundary for identifying high risk cases is located. The second trimester system used at our hospital research site, and many others, offers a 65 per cent detection at the price of a 5 per cent false positive rate.

Technical advances such as OSCAR make possible improved risk management, in this case screening which is both more accurate and speedier. However, such advances do not provide solutions to moral dilemmas, for example those entailed in deciding which forms of genetic abnormality make foetuses abortable. Moreover, anyone concerned with the imperfect prediction of uncommon events must work in an unfavourable probabilistic climate. Researchers attempting to improve Down's syndrome screening have to predict an event, the birth of babies with Down's syndrome, which occurs, in the absence of intervention, only about 1 time in 700 in the present population. This low underlying incidence means that a false positive rate of only 1 per cent (the probability of a woman screening positive given that the baby does not have Down's syndrome) will still yield seven false screen positives for every correctly identified case (a probability of 1 : 8 that the baby has Down's syndrome, given that the woman screened positive).

Amniocentesis

As already noted, women at our hospital research site might be offered amniocentesis either as their initial test, or if their serum screening result caused them to be classified into the higher risk group.

Amniocentesis involves extraction of amniotic fluid via a needle. Foetal cells are cultured, and the presence of chromosomal conditions identified directly. The test provides highly accurate results, although a small proportion of errors occur when maternal rather than foetal cells are mistakenly cultured. With respect to Down's syndrome and other chromosomal abnormalities, therefore, amniocentesis more or less banishes uncertainty and its probabilistic complications. The price paid at our hospital research site involved acceptance of intrusive procedure, a longer delay for test results (up to three weeks as against one week for serum screening) and a possibly increased risk of miscarriage.

The incidence of miscarriages resulting from amniocentesis is commonly assessed as 1–1.5 per cent (Tabor *et al.*, 1986), but declines with practice (MRC, 1977), a point which doctors involved in our research sometimes emphasised during hospital consultations, as will be seen in Chapter 7. Moreover, some experts maintain that the overall rate of amniocentesis-induced miscarriage is substantially less than 1 per cent (Sicherman *et al.*, 1995). The estimate of the risk of miscarriage entails second-order uncertainty about the accuracy of inductively estimated probabilities. Small increases in the low, but locally variable, background incidence of miscarriages cannot be easily measured.

Given the correlational, non-experimental nature of the evidence, the increased miscarriage rate associated with amniocentesis may not be caused by the procedure. However, the standard estimate of 1–2 per cent additional risk has become codified into medical knowledge and practice. Throughout the book, we will focus on this perceived risk simply because it was accepted as such by doctors, midwives and pregnant women. Whether epidemiologically warranted or not, the belief that amniocentesis increased the risk of miscarriage provided one of the grounds on which genetic screening/testing decisions were made.

Robinson (1996, p. 51) dismisses the putative 1–2 per cent increased risk as 'small', but pregnant women do not usually take this view (see Chapter 5). A small risk to one person may be unacceptably high to another, depending upon their background expectations and their evaluation of the adverse event in question.

Given the high ratio of false to true positives associated with serum screening (see Table 0.2), a strategy of offering amniocentesis to women who screen positive would result in a substantial ratio of miscarried healthy foetuses to foetuses with Down's syndrome which are detected and aborted (Spencer and Carpenter, 1985) if the true rate of amniocentesis-induced miscarriages was around 1.5 per cent. These authors estimated that screening strategies which used combinations of maternal age and serum screening levels as criteria for recommending amniocentesis would yield two or more miscarried, genetically normal foetuses for each abortion of a foetus with Down's syndrome. They note (p. 1942) that *'little comment has been made concerning the prevalence of false positives'* resulting from these strategies, which have become established as routine in maternity hospitals. Rapp (1999, p. 1) has described prenatal diagnosis as *'one of the most routinized of the new reproductive technologies'*. Although it has not, as of the year 2000, fully acquired this status in the UK, its imminent acceptance as unproblematic may be anticipated (see Chapter 1).

The genetic screening/testing risk escalator

We have used the metaphorical term *'risk escalator'* (Heyman and Henriksen, 1998b, pp. 95–103) to point up some dynamic features of preventative systems. These dynamics are found when measures of increasing intensity, associated with both higher personal and treatment costs and greater preventative efficacy, can be applied to the prevention of a type of risk.

Risk escalators can travel up or down. They move downwards towards less intense interventions which, typically, offer less safety, but cost less, entail less serious side-effects, and disrupt personal autonomy to a smaller degree. Their downward movement is powered by negative feedback insofar as more intense interventions reduce risk, thereby making weaker preventative strategies more acceptable. Upward escalators, in contrast, provide increasing levels of safety, at the price of more intense interventions. Their upward movement is fuelled by positive feedback insofar as preventative actions lower down the escalator increase risk, through unintended side-effects, and so trigger more intense interventions. The genetic screening/testing system may be viewed as a risk escalator with three levels above the ground of no intervention, namely serum screening, amniocentesis and termination. The risk escalator may move up or down, depending upon whether a woman screens positive or negative. The dynamics of the upward risk escalator arise because a screen positive makes it harder for a woman to decline amniocentesis, whilst a positive diagnosis from amniocentesis makes it more difficult for her to reject pregnancy termination. Conversely, a screen negative carries a woman downwards, making it harder for her to subsequently request amniocentesis than if she had not been screened.

Women who screen positive for Down's syndrome are faced with the choice of living with a higher risk status for several months or undergoing amniocentesis, which carries with it the perceived risk of miscarrying a healthy foetus. Only 20 per cent of these women decline this next step (Dawson *et al.*, 1993; the Northern Genetics Service, 1998). Those who receive a positive amniocentesis result at our hospital research site have to choose between knowingly bringing a baby with Down's syndrome into the world or accepting a late abortion. One study found that only half of the 26 per cent of women who stated that they would decline to terminate a pregnancy after a positive amniocentesis actually did so (Santalahti *et al.*, 1999). In each case, a positive result makes it more difficult for women not to proceed to the next level of the risk escalator. Conversely, women who screen negative for Down's syndrome, and find themselves classified as at low risk, have to discount this assessment if they subsequently opt for amniocentesis. Doctors at our research site considered that women who screened negative hardly ever requested amniocentesis, although, as we shall see in Chapter 7, they were sometimes explicitly offered this option.

Risk management systems for Down's syndrome

Maternity service providers seeking to offer women the opportunity to prevent the birth of children with Down's syndrome need to put together packages of screening/testing options, and to develop means of helping women and their families to make informed choices from the menus provided. The design of such a system requires specification of the tests to be offered to women of different ages, and of a means for communicating to them some or all of the probabilistic complexities discussed above. The specification of a system must be distinguished analytically from its operation, since, in complex organisational settings, services do not always conform in practice to official plans.

Variation in prenatal genetic screening/testing policy

National frameworks for screening policy vary substantially even in historically close, culturally similar Western societies. These variations reflect wider differences in societal values. For example, in Ireland, with its strong Catholic tradition, abortion is illegal, genetic screening/testing is not offered, and children with Down's syndrome are simply accepted. In the USA, in contrast, women aged over 35 are routinely offered invasive diagnostic tests such as amniocentesis. In Britain, compromise and local decision-making reign supreme. The genetic screening/testing system which a woman encounters depends upon a postcode lottery. In NE England and Cumbria, serum screening was, in 1997, made universally available, regardless of age, to 19 000 women attending nine maternity centres, whilst selective age-related screening was offered to 36 000 women at six centres (Northern Genetics Service, 1998). The proportions actually screened at centres offering universal screening varied between 31 per cent and 73 per cent, whilst hospitals with discretionary policies screened between 5 and 25 per cent of their populations of pregnant women. The Northern Genetics Service (1998) found that the uptake of serum screening in hospitals offering it universally was unrelated to maternal age, the main identified risk factor for Down's syndrome. A similar finding in our own study of a selective hospital is discussed in Chapter 5.

Hospitals also vary in their strategies for informing pregnant women about their genetic screening/testing options. Some utilise non-medical, trained genetic counsellors (Rapp, 1995). Some, as at our hospital research site, rely on hospital doctors giving necessarily brief advice during routine appointments. Others give midwives this role, as at a hospital which neighboured our research site, and which offered universal genetic screening. The establishment and maintenance of a specific screening/testing system requires a substantial organisational and professional investment. Such systems are continually affected by wider changes such as creeping routinisation and technical advances, such as those outlined above.

Those responsible for the operation of a preventative system are required to balance responsiveness to wider shifts against the need for organisational stability. Maintenance of a state of quasi-stable equilibrium may be assisted by the cultivation of a degree of organisational isolation. Senior doctors whom we asked about the matter were quick to assert that they did not know about the prenatal genetic screening/testing set-up in the neighbouring hospital.

Maternal genetic screening/testing at the hospital research site

Our hospital research site offers genetic screening/testing for Down's syndrome and other chromosomal conditions to women aged about 35 and over, and to those with a personal or family history of the condition. Some younger women without such a history were also offered genetic tests, as we shall see in Chapter 3. It will also be shown that, in practice, some women aged 35 and over slip through the net, and are not offered any form of genetic test. All women are seen by a hospital doctor, either a consultant or registrar, who takes the main responsibility for providing women with advice about genetic screening and testing. This topic is discussed in only 10 per cent of consultations at the hospital, according to our survey, with the topic raised first by the doctor in four-fifths of these consultations (see Chapter 3).

Maternal serum screening is carried out in our hospital in the 16th week of pregnancy, and amniocentesis, as the first test, at 14–16 weeks, as stated above. The results of serum screening and amniocentesis are returned after one and up to three weeks respectively. Women whose serum screening results lead to them being categorised as at higher risk of a Down's syndrome birth are offered a follow-up amniocentesis. The Northern Genetics Service uses a probability of 1:200 to differentiate higher and lower risk screening results. Women in the higher risk group are given their estimated probability of bearing a baby with Down's syndrome. The remainder are simply told that they are at low risk of this outcome. With respect to the higher risk group, at least, this policy meets the recommendation of Wald and Hackshaw (1997) that women should be given as precise risk information as possible. Wald and Hackshaw cite evidence (Haddow, Palomaki and Knight, 1992; Wald *et al.*, 1992) that women's decisions about accepting amniocentesis are influenced by the probability levels they are given after serum screening, with higher levels generating greater acceptance.

Overall, 80 per cent of women who receive a higher risk serum screening result accept amniocentesis (Dawson *et al.*, 1993; Northern Genetics Service, 1998), as already noted. In the small proportion of cases in which Down's syndrome is detected through the latter test, a pregnancy termination is offered. Because of the time-lags involved, women who have serum screening followed by amniocentesis may be offered an abortion late in their pregnancy, at 20 weeks. At this stage, the termination process used at the hospital requires a woman to go through a full labour in order to give birth to a dead baby (see the section on 'Late Termination' in Chapter 5). It should not be assumed, however, that late terminations will necessarily cause women and their families more emotional distress than earlier ones.

Women may be guided through the genetic screening/testing maze, summarised in Figure 3.1, in Chapter 3, in various ways, as discussed above. In our hospital, doctors advised selected women during the hospital consultation which all received. These discussions lasted for, on average, about seven minutes. Doctors freely admitted that they developed their own individual procedures for explaining the issues surrounding genetic screening/testing, that they lacked training, and that they needed further guidance about how risk information should be communicated, as found in several studies (Green, 1994; Smith *et al.*, 1995; Sadler, 1997).

Despite their crucial role in the care of pregnant women, some midwives at our hospital felt disempowered by the advent of genetic screening/testing. One stated that *'our role here has eroded. We are not a midwives' clinic anymore. It is a doctor-centred clinic.'* This shift in control was underpinned by a division of labour in which risk expertise was treated as exclusively medical. As one pregnant midwife put it:

Pregnant midwife: *The consultant will talk about statistics, and will tell you actually how much at risk you are from having a Down's syndrome, and maybe what risk you are from having a miscarriage with the amniocentesis, things like that. I don't actually give them statistics. Usually the doctors pull a chart off the wall and show them all the statistics and everything.* (Shirley, midwife, aged 34, 20 weeks, no genetic tests)

However, other midwives with whom we discussed this issue informally, maintained that they played a substantial role in advising pregnant women about genetic screening/testing. They identified a power struggle between themselves and doctors over ownership of this overlapping professional boundary. Doctors whom we asked about the appropriateness of midwives providing risk advice considered that they could, in principle, provide probabilistic information, but that many lacked the necessary education. They also pointed out that some women obtained screening privately after a brief discussion with the midwife. Doctors felt that they sometimes had to pick up the pieces if a woman screened positive.

Doctors themselves obtained their statistics from the table provided by the Northern Genetics Service. They questioned their own competence as experts in risk communication. Consultants indicated in informal discussion that they would have preferred to hand over their information-giving function to trained genetic counsellors, and to offer genetic screening to all women, but were unable to obtain funding for this service. Workload constraints prevented hospital doctors from advising more than a small proportion of women. In consequence, they could not offer genetic tests more widely.

The division of labour between doctors and midwives varies between hospitals. As already noted, other hospitals, locally and nationally, are able to offer universal genetic screening because they rely on midwives

Table 0.3   Two views of risk elements – adapted from Heyman, Henriksen and Maughan (1998)

Risk viewed as referencing natural phenomena	Risk viewed as referencing knowledge
Event	Category
Adversity	Value
Probability	Expectation
Externally defined time-scale	Time-frame

to provide genetic information. Thus, hospital policy towards the provision of risk information influences the operational scope of screening systems, and is bound up with locally negotiated patterns of interprofessional relationships.

Risk knowledge

In this section, we will outline a framework for the analysis of risk (Heyman, 1998; Heyman, Henriksen and Maughan, 1998) which will be drawn upon throughout the book. Table 0.3 offers two contrasting perspectives on risk, which can be viewed as referencing, firstly, a natural phenomenon, and, secondly, a social resource.

The treatment of risk as a natural phenomenon underlies one standard definition of risk as *'the probability that a particular adverse event occurs during a stated time period, or results from a particular challenge'* (the Royal Society, 1992, p. 2). In contrast, the approach to risk as a social resource treats it as referencing knowledge through culturally mediated projection onto the external world of uncertainty about a negatively valued event category.

Risk judgements are compounded from the four elements shown in Table 0.3. From the perspective summarised in the second column, on which the material in this book is based, the identification of a type of event, for example Down's syndrome, requires an implicit, prior act of classification. This act focuses selective attention on the category in question, maximising its distinctiveness, whilst de-emphasising both differences within the category (Tajfel, 1982) and other events which might have merited preventative consideration. The next chapter will be concerned solely with the question of how Down's syndrome is constituted, homogenised and highlighted as a risk for pregnant women.

Adversity, the second risk ingredient shown in Table 0.3, may be treated as a property of events, as in the Royal Society definition, or as a projection of value judgements. Such projections, which transform probabilities into risks, stifle debate because they cause negativity to be experienced as a property of events rather than of ways of thinking about them. The role of value judgements about Down's syndrome in women's decision-making about genetic tests will be discussed in Chapter 4 in the section on *'Value Judgements and Decision-Making'*.

Probability, like value, can be thought of as a property of events, as in the Royal Society definition, or as the projection of a degree of uncertainty about a future or otherwise unknown event. The implicit act of projection entailed by probability statements can be seen most clearly when they refer to contingencies which have already occurred, but which are not definitively known. The genetic status of the foetus is already determined before a woman is tested. The probabilistic nature of this status only arises because it is not certainly known. When risk experts inform a woman of 'her' maternal age-related risk, they simply transfer inductive knowledge about a sub-population to that woman, maintaining the useful *'fiction'* (Reichenbach, 1949) that aggregate properties of a category can be attributed to each of the individuals within it. Knowledge changes alter risks, as when a woman undergoes amniocentesis, and the probability that her baby has Down's syndrome shifts towards either virtually 1 or 0. Unless probability is reframed as the projection of uncertainty, such changes will suggest, paradoxically, that an unknown event can be changed simply and solely by learning more about it.

The reframing of probability as degree of uncertainty is discussed in the section on 'The Probability Heuristic' in Chapter 4. This heuristic differs from those now proliferating in academic psychology (Gigerenzer, Todd and the ABC Research Group, 1999) which refer to lay, rule-of-thumb simplification of complex phenomena. In contrast, the probability heuristic is embedded in scientific discourse itself, generating the taken-for-granted realities which lay people may further simplify. Inductive probabilistic thinking predicts future events which result from complex causal processes by categorising them, and then attributing empirically observed properties of the category to individual members (Heyman, Henriksen and Maughan, 1998). This reduction in the epistemological status of inductive scientific predictions requires lay probabilistic reasoning, for example, prediction from a small number of immediately available cases (Tversky and Kahneman, 1973), to be, in turn, further demoted, to the level of heuristics about heuristics.

Finally, the *'stated time period'* mentioned in the Royal Society (1992) definition of risk, cited above, begs the question of who 'states' these temporal boundaries. We will show, in Chapter 5, that women contemplating the risk of Down's syndrome adopt widely differing time frames. One woman might focus on the immediate trauma of a late termination, whilst another might worry about the biographically distant future, weighing up the impact on their other children's lives of looking after an adult with Down's syndrome after the parents have died. Women's decisions about genetic screening and testing can only be understood in relation to the time frames which they adopted, and cannot be externally *stated* or objectively delineated.

The above analysis should not be read as supporting a relativistic approach to risk. Lupton (1999a,b) has noted sociological confusion about whether risks are to be considered as real phenomena or as social constructions. She has pointed out a previously unremarked distinction between 'cultural/symbolic', 'governmentality' and 'risk society' approaches to the relationship between risk and society, based on the work of Douglas, Foucault and Beck respectively. The cultural/symbolic approach focuses on the relationship between ideas about risk and wider cultural belief systems. The governmentality approach treats risk beliefs as elements in a system of societal control which requires individuals, including pregnant women, to monitor their own behaviour preventatively. The risk society approach sees risk-consciousness as triggered by the accumulation of unwanted side-effects of technological progress.

These three approaches complement each other, at least partially. All can be usefully applied to analysis of genetic/screening testing systems. The operation of these systems is predicated on cultural value judgements about the adversity of the birth of babies with chromosomal abnormalities. They control the behaviour of pregnant women by shaping and heightening their risk consciousness. And, as with every new technology, they are accompanied by suspicion of side-effects, in this case the possibly increased risk of miscarriage associated with amniocentesis.

Although complementary, the three approaches distinguished by Lupton are founded on different epistemological assumptions. The cultural/symbolic and governmentality approaches adopt a social constructionist stance towards risk, although Douglas insists that the dangers underlying societal risk responses, for example low life expectancy in impoverished societies, *'are only too horribly real'* (Douglas, 1994, p. 29). Beck's analysis, in contrast, has been criticised as presuming that risks exist independently of cultural understanding (Wynne, 1996).

The analysis of risk as a complex construct, given above, precludes 'sterile polarisation' between 'real' physical-biological processes and 'unreal' social constructions (Wynne, 1996, p. 44). Selection of consequences for risk concern, judgements about adversity and the setting of time boundaries are predicated inescapably on social values. Inductively based judgements about probability, the most apparently factual element in the risk compound, depend, as argued above, upon a simplifying heuristic which embeds the ecological fallacy into scientific reasoning about complex phenomena, and allows many partial truths to be generated from the same data. This demotion of inductive probabilities challenges the dichotomy, jealously guarded in technological societies, between 'science' and 'non-science', threatening the foundation of their rationality. Inductively derived probabilities offer neither reality nor social construction, but crude simplification of complexity which the current stock of knowledge cannot unravel more adequately.

A becoming modesty is required about the prognostic power of risk analysis which offers a useful but crude, simplified glimpse of the future, based on value presumption, selectivity, attribution of aggregate properties to individuals and the dissection of time. We do not share the unalloyed enthusiasm expressed in the following quotation.

The revolutionary idea that defines the boundary between modern times and the past is the mastery of risk: the notion that the future is more than the whim of the gods and that men and women are not passive before nature (Bernstein, 1996, p. 1).

In the pages that follow, we will explore the presentation, by hospital doctors playing the role of risk experts, of the simplified vision of the future which risk analysis supplies, and of the complex responses of its intended beneficiaries, pregnant women.

Research methodology

This section will briefly summarise the main methodological features of the research around which the present book has been written. Data collection methods and then sampling will be briefly outlined.

Methods

Fieldwork was carried out between 1995 and 1997 in a large maternity hospital within Tyne and Wear. The initial aim of the study was to explore women's perceptions of risk in pregnancy, using a grounded theory approach (Strauss and Corbin, 1990). Women were interviewed in the hospital by the second author, a trained midwife, with interviews lasting from 45 to 150 minutes. Interviews were organised around open-ended questions about women's pregnancy experiences, concerns, reactions to professional advice and perceptions of their prospects. The risk of Down's syndrome, worry about genetic screening/testing, and a related concern about maternal age, emerged as important issues for pregnant women, particularly, but not exclusively, for those aged 35 and over. The research was then directed towards this issue. Subsequent interviews were undertaken mainly with the older age group, although a sample of very young mothers was also interviewed for purposes of contrast. Some older pregnant midwives were also interviewed, so that the insights of people who had changed role from practitioner to service user could be drawn upon (Heyman and Henriksen, 1998a, pp. 53–5). Information about the sample is provided below.

Analysis of these interviews generated further questions, which were explored through additional data collection. A large questionnaire survey of pregnant women at 34 or more weeks' gestation was undertaken, in order to investigate factors associated with being offered and accepting genetic tests; and to assess the contextual question of women's age norms about parenting. A sample of hospital consultations was tape-recorded, and analysed qualitatively. Where possible, follow-up interviews were carried out with these women, so that their understanding of the hospital consultation could be related to what had been said. Hospital doctors and midwives were interviewed about their views of the genetic screening/testing system. Finally, feedback about findings was obtained from doctors and midwives, through both informal group and individual discussion.

Interviews were taped and fully transcribed. Permission to carry out the research was given by the local medical ethics committee. Women received an information sheet which emphasised the voluntary and confidential nature of research participation. All the names of research participants have been changed. In order to protect doctors' identity we have not indicated whether a consultant or registrar is being quoted. For the same reason, we refer to all 13 doctors, two female and 11 male, who participated in the research in gender-neutral language, substituting the term [the doctor] for male and female pronouns in quotations. Quotations involving pregnant women are referenced in terms of her age, the information source, her doctor if a genetic consultation is being referenced, her gestation and her eventual screening/testing decision. Where a quotation comes from a pregnant midwife, this has been noted.

The research samples

Information about the research samples is provided in Table 0.4.

Women were surveyed towards the end of their pregnancy, at a mean gestation of 35 weeks, and would have known the results of any genetic tests. Similarly, women were mostly interviewed during their pregnancy, either after they had declined to be genetically screened or tested, or had received their results. (Three women were interviewed post-partum, and one was intending to use amniocentesis in a future,

Table 0.4 The research sample

Data collection method	Number in final sample	Response rate	Age range	Number aged >= 35
Interviews with pregnant women, excluding midwives	35	100%	14–41	16
Interviews with pregnant midwives	6	100%	31–42	4
Survey of pregnant women	1552	97%	15–43	109
Transcription of hospital consultations[1]	16	100%	25–46	13
Follow-up interviews after hospital consultation[2]	10	63%	25–46	9
Interviews with hospital doctors	11	100%	–	–
Interviews with midwives	5	100%	–	–

[1] Four additional consultations were taped subsequently, but not intensively analysed.
[2] Two of these ten women, who underwent amniocentesis with a positive and negative result respectively, received two follow-up interviews before and after they received their results.

planned pregnancy.) The data, therefore, provide a mainly retrospective perspective. However (see next paragraph) women whose hospital consultation had been recorded and transcribed were interviewed, where possible, shortly after. This combined method offers a more dynamic view of the genetic/screening process, and generated some of the richest data.

As can be seen in Table 0.4, high response rates were generally obtained, perhaps as a result of the good will with which the NHS is still regarded in British society. A somewhat higher proportion of women declined to be interviewed after their hospital consultation had been taped. This sample of ten women includes two respondents who underwent amniocentesis and were interviewed twice, before and after they had received the results. One of these women received a negative test result, whilst the other underwent a termination following the diagnosis of foetal Down's syndrome (see Chapter 5). The questionnaires were given out in the maternity hospital. Very few women refused to accept them, and a surprisingly high 97 per cent returned them.

Structure of the book

The book will first explore, in Chapter 1, the constitution, at our hospital research site, of the birth of a child with Down's syndrome as a risk warranting the concern of women aged roughly 35 and over. We will show that this contingency is constituted as a risk by the genetic screening/testing system in operation at our hospital research site, which highlights it as a difficult to manage problem. Risk status is acquired through socially organised concern about the occurrence of a future or otherwise unknown event, not through its inherent properties. Lacking the benefit of probabilistic analysis, events simply occur or do not occur. The reframing of probability as externalised uncertainty leaves no room for risks to exist independently of somebody thinking about them.

Future or otherwise unknown events only become risks when social groups classify and worry about them. The organisational processes which transform a contingency into a risk will be elucidated in Chapter 1 through a comparison between the risk of Down's syndrome and the non-risks of spina bifida and stillbirths. The non-risk status of spina bifida arises from the routinisation of screening scans, not the lack of problems such as false positives and negatives with the procedure, whilst the non-risk status, for most pregnant women, of stillbirths derives from their unpredictability.

The wider issue of being 'old' in relation to pregnancy will be considered in Chapter 2. We will argue that women calibrate their ages using multiple biographical clocks which measure maternal age in different ways, for example, in relation to their fitness, careers and length of marriage. Women judge their medically defined genetic age in the context of these other chronologies.

Chapter 3 will be concerned with the processes governing the offer of genetic tests for Down's syndrome. We will show that women were more likely to be offered genetic tests, regardless of their age, if they were concerned about the health of their baby for any reason. Hospital doctors readily acknowledged that they might offer genetic tests in order to reassure women whose anxiety they sensed. Ironically, an anxiety-provoking procedure was used for intended psycho-therapeutic purposes. The genetic screening/testing system at our hospital research site, thus operated as a hybrid between the two modes postulated by Castel (1996), with doctors both screening a population and responding, in a fashion, to the needs of individuals.

Chapters 4 and 5 will explore, in some detail, women's decision-making about genetic screening/testing. Their value judgements about Down's syndrome, miscarriage and abortion, and their probabilistic reasoning will be discussed in Chapter 4. Chapter 5 will focus on the different ways in which pregnant women take account of time in their risk appraisals, and on their genetic screening/testing decisions. These two chapters, together with Chapter 1, will work through the four elements of risk as a social resource summarised in Table 0.3, namely categories, values, probabilities and time frames.

The next two chapters will explore, again in some detail, risk communication. Chapter 6 covers the discussion of the pre-test risk of Down's syndrome and, where mentioned, other chromosomal conditions. Chapter 7 analyses discussion of the changes to the risk picture which result from genetic screening and testing, particularly the effect of serum screening on a woman's individual probability of giving birth to a baby with Down's syndrome, and the risk of miscarriage arising from amniocentesis. We will show that, despite doctors' best efforts to depict risk as neutrally as possible, its representation was coloured by subtle but critical differences of interpretation and presentation.

Finally, the Conclusion will briefly draw out a number of implications of the study for social scientific understanding of the operation of screening systems, even sketching some practical implications for genetic counselling. We make no claims about the typicality of the screening system under examination. On the contrary, we would argue that, particularly in the absence of national or international standardisation, every concrete realisation of such a system takes its own organisational form. Nevertheless, detailed examination of one screening system can generate propositions about their working which may have a wider significance.

1
The Constitution of Down's Syndrome as a Risk Entity

Introduction

In this chapter, we will consider the constitution of Down's syndrome as a risk entity worthy of selective attention, and demanding rational decision-making. We will show that the hospital doctors who managed, and were most committed to, the genetic screening/testing system took the status of Down's syndrome as a risk management problem for granted. The views of pregnant women and midwives, in contrast, varied considerably. The questions which they raised subverted the rationality of the preventative system for Down's syndrome by challenging the unquestioned presuppositions upon which it was predicated. These presuppositions are: that individual cases of Down's syndrome can be considered equivalent in probabilistic calculations; that the occurrence of the condition is predictable and preventable; and that prevention raises dilemmas which preclude the identification of a treatment of choice.

We will argue that a contingency only becomes a risk when it is deemed to have these properties; and that the status of Down's syndrome as a risk reflects the organisation of health services around a prevailing stock of knowledge rather than intrinsic attributes of the condition. The argument will be documented through a contrast of the risk status of Down's syndrome, firstly, with that of spina bifida, the detection of which via screening scans is now routinised in the UK; and, secondly, with that of stillbirths which were not screened for. These last two contingencies did not possess the combination of attributes required for elevation to risk status, namely problematic preventability.

The classification of Down's syndrome as an event

Considerable knowledge of both the genetic antecedents and consequences of Down's syndrome has accumulated in recent years. This
knowledge can be differentiated from that available for conditions such
as ulcerative colitis, which can be defined relatively precisely in terms of
their symptoms, but whose aetiology is ill understood; and for conditions
which cannot be clearly defined in terms of either their manifestation or
their causes, for instance schizophrenia. Since both the aetiology and
consequences of Down's syndrome are well understood, we might expect
to find the constitution of Down's syndrome as an event reasonably
unproblematic. However, because of its variable symptomology, Rapp
(1988, p. 150) has described the term Down's syndrome as an *'iconic
description'* which directs attention away from clinically and humanly
significant differences. Such selective attention results inexorably from
the nomothetic classification of complex phenomena (Tajfel, 1982).

Since no common, unvaried consequence of trisomy 21 other than
a highly variable degree of intellectual impairment has been identified
(Shapiro, 1997), the nature of Down's syndrome can only be established through comparison of the average profiles of those with and
without the condition. This type of thinking can be related to the prevailing epidemiological approach which identifies trends through comparisons of sub-populations, and then applies them, via an unexamined
conceptual leap, to individuals within observer-defined categories
(Rose, 1985). Disturbed lung growth (Schloo, Vawter and Reid, 1991),
congenital heart disease (Marino, 1993), obesity (Prasher, 1995), liver
disease (Ruchelli *et al.*, 1990) depression (Cooper and Collacott, 1994),
child hyperactivity (Pueschel, Bernier and Pezzullo, 1991) and many
other conditions occur with greater prevalence in the population of
people with Down's syndrome. In epidemiologically oriented risk societies, such evidence may be taken to demonstrate that individuals carry
with them the higher or lower risk associated with a category to which
they have been assigned.

This way of thinking suffers from two important limitations. Firstly,
it discounts the possibility that some, at least, of the identified risks may
result from the impact of the iconography of the allegedly dangerous
condition on quality of life. For example, the increased prevalence of
depression in adults, and of hyperactivity in children, with Down's Syndrome might be explained in terms of frustration arising from poorer
life chances which, in turn, result from negative cultural attitudes to
people with the condition.

Secondly, knowledge of comparative frequencies of specific adverse events in observer-defined sub-populations does not tell us about individual patterns of occurrence (Rose, 1985), except in the limiting case where all the individuals in the marked category experience the adverse event whilst no individuals in the comparison group do so. (This point is discussed in the section on *'The Probability Heuristic'* in Chapter 4.) In this case, perfect prediction would have been achieved, and risk analysis would not be required. In theory, a string of comparisons showing people with Down's syndrome to be at higher risk of a range of health problems would be found if a small minority suffered most of these conditions, whilst others experienced no problems other than a greater or lesser degree of intellectual disability. Knowledge about patterns of health problems cannot be derived from the studies of individual conditions which our highly specialised medical system tends to generate.

One holistic study (McGrother and Marshall, 1990) of the range of conditions experienced by children with Down's syndrome noted in passing that nearly half did not suffer from any recorded medical complications whatsoever, whilst the other 56 children faced a total of 71 serious or fatal health problems. Future advances in genetic knowledge about trisomy 21 might enable sub-groups with different probabilities of experiencing various health problems to be differentiated (see the Introduction). The present categorisation of babies with Down's syndrome as at increased risk of a range of medical complications depends upon the limitations of current knowledge which does not permit finer sub-categorisations to be developed for predictive purposes. Such historically delimited disease entities then become associated with a cultural iconography, as already noted.

This discounting of differences should not be regarded as scandalous, but as an inevitable price to be paid for generalisation. Once the differences within a category have been backgrounded, membership can be related probabilistically to its antecedents and consequences through inductive inference from epidemiological evidence. The resulting nomothetic knowledge can be used to obtain a crude picture of individual futures which goes beyond what could be achieved with the given stock of specific causal knowledge. Challenges to the assumption of homogeneity subvert the status of such arduously acquired, but limited, prognostic power. An epidemiology of Down's syndrome which differentially predicted the probability of mild versus serious intellectual disability, and of major, as against minor, physical complications would require a totally new empirical base, and would generate a new risk analysis. Not surprisingly, hospital doctors did not undermine the credentials of their own expertise by raising questions about the classificatory schema for Down's syndrome, as we will see below.

Qualitative analysis allows the iconography of Down's syndrome to be explored with reference to the perceptions of both pregnant women and health professionals.

Women's views of Down's syndrome as an event

Once a category has been embedded in a culture, it will become linked to culturally derived imagery which then may be seen as inevitably and invariably associated with the homogenised condition. As one woman, who had decided with her husband to terminate the life of her baby after Down's syndrome was diagnosed (see Chapter 5), put it:

> **Pregnant woman:** *I mean you can't get away from the fact that they are ... I mean their eyes come out, they have floppy tongues ... It's just endless.* (Mary, aged 46, interview after pregnancy termination, 17 weeks, amniocentesis)

This couple's decision, taken with deep regret and uncertainty, to terminate the pregnancy cannot be divorced from the imagery which they both associated with the category of people with Down's syndrome, and then applied to all present and future members of that category.

Only two of the 41 women who were interviewed mentioned differences within the Down's syndrome category. One of these anomalous respondents had, unlike most health professionals or pregnant women, directly experienced the life of a relative with the condition.

> **Woman anticipating pregnancy:** *I think I would have thought of Down's syndrome because I have got an uncle. But I have always been very much aware, although he was a really healthy Down's syndrome, he did not have any heart problems.* (Yvonne, aged 35, interview, not pregnant, intending to choose amniocentesis)

Despite recognising differences within the category of Down's syndrome, this woman, who was planning to become pregnant, had definitely decided to opt for amniocentesis and termination if necessary. The second woman who recognised differences within the Down's syndrome category also eventually chose amniocentesis, on the grounds that she and her husband were too old to look after a baby with Down's syndrome over the longer term. But she vehemently rejected the homogenisation of people with the condition.

> **Pregnant woman:** *And it doesn't help, again, people making comments like, what he* [acquaintance] *just said, 'You could be changing someone's nappy at 21.' I mean, not all Down's syndrome are like that, are they? I have seen them walking around the town. And, apart from their visual looks, they are very intelligent, some of them.* (Marietta, aged 39, interview after taped hospital consultation [Laughton], 12 weeks, amniocentesis)

No other research participant treated Down's syndrome as other than a homogenous condition. A woman quoted by Rothman (1988, p. 99) rejected abortion for babies with this condition on the grounds that *'even the term "Down's syndrome" implies the whole spectrum of possibilities from mildly retarded to severely so, and a similar spectrum of physical ills'*. Lippman-Hand and Fraser (1979b) found that parental awareness of the variable manifestation of genetic abnormalities complicated their decision-making, as they could not evaluate the severity of consequences even if the probability of a condition could be well-specified. Hence, subversion of the medically legitimated diagnostic classification system undermined the rationality of decisions based on risk analysis.

Medical views of Down's syndrome as an event

Doctors' views about the nature of Down's syndrome are, inevitably, coloured by their professional socialisation, as well as wider cultural attitudes and variable personal influences. In Western societies, at least, obstetricians assess Down's syndrome as a more adverse event than do the general public (Drake, Reid and Marteau, 1996). This pessimistic perspective may affect service provision in two ways: indirectly, by providing the impetus for the development of screening systems which draw selective attention to the prevention of Down's syndrome (see next section); and directly, through colouring doctors' presentation of the condition to pregnant women.

The most recent information pack provided by the Northern Genetics Service (1997) for health professionals giving advice to pregnant women about chromosomal abnormalities contains a supplementary leaflet, not present in the 1995 version. The information pack comments that:

professionals tend to omit the positive aspects and concentrate upon the abnormalities and difficulties associated with Down's syndrome. It is probably better to establish the degree of familiarity which concerned individuals have with the condition, then allow them to ask the actual questions for which they wish to obtain an answer – rather than to report a list of medical facts.

However, the next part of the leaflet lists the many medical complications associated with Down's syndrome.

Doctors generally said little or nothing about the symptomology of Down's syndrome in consultations about prenatal genetic screening and testing, progressing immediately to a discussion of the probability of this undefined condition, as will be shown in Chapter 6. The following interview extract suggests that the doctor quoted took a common understanding of Down's syndrome for granted.

> **Interviewer:** *Do you talk to them* [pregnant women] *about Down's syndrome, about what Down's syndrome is?*
> **Doctor:** *No, I don't actually . . . interesting. And yet, of course, that is addressed in the film* [provided for pregnant women], *isn't it? Perhaps I should do.* (Bell, interview)

The expression of surprise suggests that this doctor had discovered an unexamined presupposition. The next doctor quoted 'assumed' that women would understand the nature of the contingency around which the hospital consultation was organised. This respondent also argued that their caseload prevented doctors from doing more than taking a common understanding of Down's syndrome for granted.

> **Interviewer:** *Do you talk about Down's syndrome?*
> **Doctor:** *No.*
> **Interviewer:** *What Down's syndrome is?*
> **Doctor:** *No. I assume that they understand, and they've read the leaflet before they came to see me, because we see about eight or nine new bookings every clinic. We don't really have time to go through this.* (Rowntree, interview)

The next medical respondent cited also believed that doctors and pregnant women shared a common understanding about the nature of Down's syndrome, but reported testing out this assumption in hospital consultations.

Interviewer: *Do you discuss Down's syndrome in your screening sessions? Do you talk about it?*
Doctor: *I ask if they understand what is meant by Down's because I don't think you should ever assume that people know. I mean, certainly, if you say trisomy 21 to them, they certainly wouldn't understand that . . . And I haven't yet come across anybody who didn't know what a Down's baby was, or what I was talking about. But, if they didn't, then, I then explain to them what the most common abnormalities were, and why we were testing.* (Green, interview)

Two features of this account should be noted. Firstly, public ignorance of the genetic cause of Down's syndrome is contrasted with public knowledge of its manifestation in the syndrome itself. Secondly, both types of knowledge are treated as unproblematic. Questions about the socially mediated expression of variable genetic blueprints are, therefore, implicitly discounted. Nevertheless, the above doctor readily acknowledged the variability of the condition in response to interview probing.

Interviewer: *And do you ever, in that discussion, talk about degrees of Down's syndrome, or do you not go that far into it?*
Doctor: *Not as a routine. It has come up a couple of times in counselling sessions that the more that the patient has asked, 'Well, how badly affected will the baby be?' And then I will lead on from there to say that a lot of Down's babies will be completely fine. You may not, you can hardly tell facially that they are Down's babies, and their intelligence may be fair to moderate. They may actually be able to lead a fairly normal life, whereas, at the other scale, you may have a completely handicapped child that is going to be dependent on you for everything for the rest of its life. But I don't do that routinely. That tends to come from them, and then I expand on it from there.* (Green, interview)

The Down's syndrome profile, public 'knowledge' of which this doctor took for granted, describes the average constellation of intellectual, health and social problems within the classified population. Despite excluding routine discussion of the nature of the condition in question, this doctor still described the transactions which took place in hospital consultations as *'counselling'*. The few discussions about the nature of Down's syndrome which we did observe in the hospital consultations will be discussed in Chapter 6, in the section on *'The Meaning of Down's Syndrome'*.

Kolker and Burke (1994, p. 51) found, in the USA, that 18 out of 23 genetic counsellors reported that they always or usually described Down's syndrome in a way which was *'tailored to the client's frequently considerable knowledge'*. Trained genetic counsellors providing longer sessions may discuss this issue more fully. However, an approach which draws upon public understanding may take for granted 'knowledge' which is itself problematic, given the iconic status of the Down's syndrome category.

Selective attention to Down's syndrome

Event classes generate an indefinitely large number of qualitatively distinct consequences. Only those which are identified can be considered for preventative action. Some of these consequences will, inevitably, be pursued more systematically than others. Even in highly medicalised Western societies, birth entails risk for both mother and baby. The risks incurred by the mother include death, unbearable pain, post-natal depression, loss of youthful appearance, infection and raised blood pressure. Babies are subject to the risk of miscarriage, stillbirth and the development of a wide range of health problems such as heart defects, limb deformities, cystic fibrosis and spina bifida.

Hospital doctors and other health professionals may emphasise the range of risks which women and their unborn babies face. Instructively, a consultant in the hospital site for one survey of women's views of maternity services raised an issue of *'acute concern'* to him, namely *'the patient's understanding of the risks involved in becoming pregnant and having a baby'* (Martin, 1992, p. 152). Schuman and Marteau (1993) concluded that obstetricians were more likely than midwives or pregnant women to regard pregnancy as a state involving risk. Rothman (1988) found that this perspective often overrode women's own feelings about genetic abnormalities, tests and abortion.

In risk societies, the very term 'risk' carries strong moral force, through the culturally reinforced imperative that risks, *ceteris paribus*, ought to be prevented. However, health-care systems cannot give equal attention to all the contingencies which affect pregnant women and their babies. Bio-medically oriented hospital systems give relatively little attention to the risk of maternal post-natal depression; or to the iatrogenic risk that high-tech preventative procedures will raise women's anxiety levels, with potentially damaging consequences for the health of the mother and baby (Lane, 1995).

As noted previously, the hospital site for our research operated a loose policy of targeting women aged 35[+] for genetic consultation with a doctor, whilst leaving the door open for younger women to receive this service. Women in the hospital catchment area lived in a health-care environment in which being 35^+ propelled them, although by no means with perfect reliability, into a group marked as needing the special attention of a doctor because of their age-related, higher risk of Down's syndrome.

Focus on Down's Syndrome entailed a selective simplification even within the sphere of chromosomal abnormalities. As we shall see, in the chapters that follow, doctors and pregnant women in our hospital research site largely treated terms such as Down's syndrome and chromosomal abnormality as equivalent. Although this was rarely explained to them, only about half the chromosomal abnormalities detected via amniocentesis involve trisomy 21, the genetic cause of Down's syndrome (Ferguson-Smith, 1983; Harper, 1991). For example, Edward's syndrome, a usually fatal condition resulting from trisomy 18, occurs with frequencies relative to Down's syndrome of $1:10$ at term, and $1:3$ at the end of the first trimester, and these prevalences are probably not age-related (Cuckle, 1997). Doctors may (with occasional exceptions, discussed in Chapter 6), have excluded consideration of chromosomal problems other than Down's syndrome because the maternal age-related statistics, supplied by the regional genetic advisory service, referenced only this condition. Moreover, consideration of these individually infrequent but cumulatively significant conditions would have greatly complicated an already complex risk picture.

We assessed the impact of this focus upon the risk of Down's syndrome on pregnant women in three different ways, through the questionnaire survey, qualitative interviews and transcripts of hospital consultations. In the survey sample, 28 per cent (29) of women aged 35 and over agreed that they were concerned about the health of their baby, compared with 17 per cent (243) of concerned women aged under 35 (chi-square = 7.3 with 1 d.f., P. < 0.01). This finding suggests that, although the risk society has penetrated the population included in our research, the majority of women, in contrast to some obstetricians, do not treat their pregnancy primarily as a risk.

Among older women who were concerned about the health of their baby, genetic issues predominated. Reasons for their concern were offered by 92 per cent (251) of worried women of all ages. Among 27 concerned respondents aged 35 and over, 70 per cent (19) were worried about foetal abnormalities, detection of problems from screening or the effects of maternal age on the baby, compared with only 31 per cent (78) of women aged less than 35 (chi-square = 21.6 with 1 d.f.,

P. < 0.0001). This finding suggests that, among risk-conscious pregnant women at our hospital research site, genetic concerns predominate in the older groups, whilst younger women worry about other problems which troubled both age groups, for example, miscarriage. However, concern about abnormalities is not a historically new phenomenon. A previous study (the Royal College of Midwives, 1966) found that 58 per cent of a sample of pregnant women mentioned fear of an abnormality, and that this fear was mentioned more frequently than any other. The risk society may have changed the ways in which its members relate to the future, seen as potentially controllable in new ways, rather than the nature of their concerns.

Our qualitative interview data uncovered more signs of risk consciousness than did the survey, with 11 out of 16 women aged over 34 having experienced significant worry about the pregnancy outcome, and Down's syndrome a major concern in 10 of these 11 cases. This discrepancy cannot be attributed to differences in the average gestational stages of the survey and interview samples, which were roughly similar. The interviews may have provided a more sensitive instrument for detecting such anxieties. One woman said that *'until I got the results of, you know, the amnio . . . it was just all worry, and I wouldn't like to go through that again now'* (Beatrice, aged 40, interview, 26 weeks, amniocentesis). A second respondent characterised her pregnancy as *'worrying . . . purely because of my age'*, and feared *'any abnormalities'* (Hilary, aged 40, interview, 23 weeks, amniocentesis).

The woman quoted below backgrounded risks other than Down's syndrome, which preoccupied her.

Interviewer: *What types of risks do you think of in pregnancy?*
Pregnant woman: *Apart from Down's?*
Interviewer: *Is that your main worry?*
Pregnant woman: *That's my main concern.*
Interviewer: *Why is that?*
Pregnant woman: *Just because of my age, and just because people say it happens when you are that age.* (Patricia, aged 37, interview, 24 weeks, serum screening)

According to the aggregate statistics supplied by the Northern Genetics Service (1995), 1:240 women of her age give birth to a baby with Down's syndrome. But she saw it as something which *'happens'* to women of her age.

Selective attention to this contingency could blot out consideration of all the many other risks which medicine links to pregnancy and birth.

Pregnant woman: *'Cos I'd said, the results* [of amniocentesis] *were supposed to have came through, and they didn't come through. And I was stressed out of me head, and I was phoning all the time . . . And I went in, and I spoke to* [hospital doctor]. *And* [doctor]*'d said to me that even if the test comes through, and it's negative, as in positive, the baby's ok, it doesn't mean that everything is ruled out. Which I expected, that. But it still came as a, 'Oh God! There still could be something wrong.'* (Lesley, aged 37, interview, 26 weeks, amniocentesis)

The hospital doctor had attempted to put this woman's anxiety about Down's syndrome in perspective by reminding her that she faced many other risks to the baby's health. But her selective attention was reinforced by the hospital screening policy itself, and the attempted reassurance widened the focus of her panic. As always in risk analysis, questions can be asked about why only some of the many possible consequences of a complex process, such as having a baby, are highlighted.

Although women did not necessarily internalise the hospital risk perspective, some needed to make a deliberate effort to think differently. One woman had consciously adopted a short time-frame in order to prevent her risk-consciousness from generating anxiety.

Pregnant midwife: *I mean, I don't look at it* [intermittent nausea] *as if I could be like this for the whole of the nine months. I mean, I know, in the back of my mind, that it could be. And, in some ways, it's* [nausea] *helped me to think I'll deal with today, you know, and I won't worry. And I think that's probably what parents have to do. I'll worry about now, you know, when they are in the cots, not whether they are going to be sniffing glue in six years' time. So it's done that, it's changed my way of thinking in that respect.* (Jackie, midwife, aged 36, interview, 14 weeks, no genetic tests)

The same respondent had recognised the connection between the availability of test procedures and selective attention to those risks which could be assessed.

Pregnant midwife: *So I did talk with* [friend], *and she was very much, and she was, well, which is true, that they can only screen for Down's and* *spina bifida, and maybe encephaly, but you don't know about birth trauma. You don't know about all those things that might be going on in there that they can't screen for.* (Jackie, midwife, aged 36, interview, 14 weeks, no genetic tests)

The health-care system, in effect, enjoined women to concentrate on those risks, and only those risks, which could be assessed and managed. Hospital consultations with older women, as will be seen in Chapters 6 and 7, were mostly organised around the management of the risk of Down's syndrome.

Doctor: *You're 38, so you are wondering about the question of Down's syndrome?* (Hazel, aged 38, hospital consultation [Crabtree], 8 weeks, serum screening)

The preventability of Down's syndrome

Risk management only becomes possible if the following two conditions are met. Firstly, cases must be identifiable, but only probabilistically. Secondly, means of prevention, in some sense, must be available. Events which cannot currently be prevented, for example residing on a planet which is struck by asteroids, may be classified technically as risks because their probability of occurrence and their adversity can be assessed. However, they attract remarkably little interest. The risks which trouble denizens of the risk society raise pragmatic concerns, as events which ought or ought not to require preventative efforts. With respect to Down's syndrome, pregnancy termination provides the only currently available method of preventing the live birth of a baby with the condition.

The link between risk consciousness and the ascription of pre-ventability is illustrated by the following pair of quotations in which a woman contrasts her anxiety level about Down's syndrome before and after having ruled out genetic tests. Initially, this woman's experience of pregnancy was dominated by her concern about the risk of Down's syndrome.

Interviewer: *So it's the practical things, it's not so much about the health of the baby?*
Pregnant woman: *No, well apart from what I say at the back of my mind, the Down's Syndrome, ehm.*
Interviewer: *Is that a big worry?*

Pregnant woman: *It was big worry when I went to the hospital. I mean, I thought about nothing else.* (Diane, aged 38, interview, 16 weeks, no genetic tests)

The above quotation well illustrates selective attention to the risk of Down's syndrome, as discussed above. However, after this respondent had decided that she could not prevent the birth of a child with Down's syndrome because she could not go through with an abortion, her attitude towards this contingency changed dramatically.

Pregnant woman: *Once I'd come to the decision not to do anything about it, I thought, 'Well, I'm not going to spend the rest of the pregnancy worrying about it, and I've made a decision.'* (Diane, aged 38, interview, 16 weeks, no genetic tests)

A future contingency which was re-classified as uncontrollable ceased, for this woman, to be a risk. This critical quotation illustrates the link between the risk status of a contingency and its perceived preventability. More broadly, it illustrates the association between risk consciousness and attitude towards the future.

The routinisation of screening scans

The routinisation of ultrasound screening scans for conditions such as spina bifida at our hospital research site contrasted with the problematisation of genetic screening/testing for Down's syndrome. We will argue below that this difference can be explained historically. Screening scans have been provided for long enough to have become accepted as a natural element in pregnancy, whilst genetic tests still retain their novel, and therefore debatable, status. This organisational difference affected the risk perceptions of women who participated in our study, since they worried far more about the risk of Down's syndrome than they did about the risks of conditions such as spina bifida which are investigated through scans.

As will be seen in Chapter 7, hospital doctors emphasised the dilemmas faced by women deciding about genetic tests, stressed that no right or wrong answers to these dilemmas could be provided, and gave women responsibility for deciding which tests, if any, to accept. In contrast, they took it for granted that women would undergo screening scans. This contrast can be seen clearly in the following quotation from a hospital consultation.

> **Doctor:** *Do you want some time alone to have a think* [about genetic test decision]?
> **Pregnant woman:** *What do you* [husband] *think?*
> **Husband:** *It's up to you.*
> **Doctor:** *I'm not pushing it on you.*
> **Pregnant woman:** *Well I think no, because, at the end of the day, if it came to it, I wouldn't want a termination anyway . . .*
> **Doctor:** *Are you happy about having a scan at 20 weeks, to make sure that there is no obvious abnormality.*
> **Pregnant woman:** *Yes.*
> **Doctor:** *You are happy about that? So we will organise for you to have a scan, a 20 week scan.* (Heather, aged 36, hospital consultation [Bell], 16 weeks, no genetic tests)

The quoted woman's main objection to genetic screening/testing, that she would not choose to terminate even if an abnormality was discovered, applied equally to diagnostic scans. The contrasting routinised and problematic status of scans and genetic screening/testing can be seen even more clearly in the next quotation.

> **Doctor:** *So I don't myself worry about people who don't have a* [serum screening/amniocentesis] *test, because our scans are good at picking up the spina bifidas, except the minor ones but they won't be devastating in terms of your baby.* (Heather, aged 36, hospital consultation [Bell], 16 weeks, no genetic tests)

Although the above doctors represented screening scan results as clear-cut, at least with respect to major conditions, other doctors pointed out their possible uncertain status, but still regarded their use as routine.

> **Doctor:** *All I would like to say to you is that there are hard signs and soft signs* [from scans]. *And what I mean by that is that there are some things that we can see, that we know are definitely associated. And there are other things that we can see on the scan sometimes, that we don't know might be associated. And there are different things that we can look for that tell us one thing or another.* (Charlotte, aged 36, hospital consultation [Fallowfield], 12 weeks, amniocentesis)

In contrast, as we shall see, doctors treated limited accuracy as a significant drawback of genetic screening. Moreover, they emphasised that the birth of a genetically abnormal foetus could only be prevented through abortion.

The routine medical status of screening scans, and their acceptance by pregnant women, can also be seen in the statistics for their take-up. Only three women out of the 1507 (97 per cent) who answered this question in our survey reported having received no scans, whilst 89 per cent (1223) indicated that they had been given two or more. The take-up rate of offered scans was 90 per cent. Some of these scans would have been intended solely for dating, but most would have been used to screen for abnormalities. Similarly, Santalahti *et al.* (1999) found, in Finland, that 85 per cent of their sample of pregnant women reported that diagnostic scans had been presented as a routine procedure. Only 22 per cent stated that serum screening had been offered in this way.

The routinisation of screening scans was powerfully portrayed in an episode of the BBC television soap opera *East Enders* (15/09/98) in which a pregnant woman, Bianca, ran out of the hospital, watched by amazed staff, because she did not wish to be scanned for spina bifida. Her family and hospital staff had assumed, without asking her, that she wished to undergo this procedure.

The woman quoted below had not realised that she could decline to be scanned.

> **Interviewer:** *Why did you decide to have the scan?*
> **Pregnant woman:** *Oh they give you them automatically, yes.*
> **Interviewer:** *You still have a choice* [if] *you want the scan.*
> **Pregnant woman:** *Oh, I didn't realise that. I thought they just give you them as a matter of fact, you know what I mean.* (Denise, aged 36, interview, 32 weeks, no genetic tests)

The ascription of the status of *'matter of fact'* to scans neatly summarises their now established, organisationally derived, routine normality. The above respondent accepted scans because she wanted to see her baby, a side benefit which may obscure their diagnostic purpose. However, if an abnormality had been detected, she might have received information which, given a choice, she would not have wished to obtain.

An incidental side benefit of the technology, that it provides them with an early moving image of the expected baby, may have obscured its diagnostic purpose.

Pregnant woman: *The scans are lovely 'cos I see all the spine, two hands, two legs, everything. And when you got the picture, it was not the same.*

Interviewer: *Did you look for those things when you went?*

Pregnant woman: *Well,* [the doctor] *was showing us. They were great. They were showing us every little bit.*

Interviewer: *Did your husband go?*

Pregnant woman: *Oh yes, me husband came. He was trying to see what sex it was, like* [laughs]. (Wendy, aged 35, 29 weeks, interview, serum screening)

The next woman quoted, a nurse who had ruled out termination in any circumstances, nicely articulated the dual diagnostic and bonding functions of screening scans.

Pregnant woman: *Well, I suppose I've contradicted myself here really, haven't I? I suppose I want to know, and I don't want to know. But, having said that, I want pictures. I want to see it, because every time, certainly, with this pregnancy as well, every time I see it, it makes it real to me that I'm having a baby.* (Elizabeth, aged 25, interview after hospital consultation [Fallowfield], 13 weeks, no genetic tests)

Doctors enjoy giving parents the pleasure of seeing their baby, and this activity lightens the grim business of risk management. For the last but one woman quoted, viewing the scan provided a means of involving the father in the birth process.

Although women and their partners enjoyed viewing the baby on the scan, its diagnostic function could generate intense anxiety.

Pregnant woman: *I could see the screen first, and then* [the doctor] *tilted the screen . . . so I couldn't see. And I thought, and that made it even more suspicious, 'Blooming heck, there's something the matter here.' And, at the end,* [the doctor] *asked the radiologist, er,* [the doctor] *couldn't find the kidneys. And* [the doctor] *says, 'Oh, it was the shadows', or something. He* [husband] *. . . thought there was something wrong, you know. And, em, I says, 'I think* [the doctor] *was just practising, just, like, having a turn.'* (Hilary, aged 40, interview, 23 weeks, amniocentesis)

The insensitivity of hospital staff, in this case, to the risk consciousness of parents waiting for the scan verdict turned their visual encounter with their baby into a negative experience.

Because doctors presented scans as unproblematic, women may not have appreciated that their use raised similar issues to those which were discussed so carefully in relation to genetic screening/testing. In particular, women who ruled out a termination in any circumstances might have felt that they did not wish to be placed in the position of knowingly bringing a baby with health problems into the world.

Ironically, doctors at our hospital research site used a number of scan indicators, for example nuchal fold thickness, as soft markers of Down's syndrome meriting discussion with parents and possible further investigation. (They had not introduced systematic use of this marker for mass screening as of February 2000, when this book went to press.) But parents were informed of their use only through a leaflet which the researchers were unable to obtain either in the maternity clinic or the antenatal ward. We do not recite this anecdote as evidence of neglect, but as an illustration of the power of routinisation. Great care was taken to inform women about prenatal genetic screening/testing, and to provide them with an explicit licence to choose from or reject the available options. In contrast, diagnostic scans had acquired the status of a normal element in pregnancy. Their use as an element in genetic screening contributed to the routinisation of this new sphere of medical surveillance.

Inevitably, comparisons of the organisational status of preventative procedures are clouded by differences in their properties. Prenatal diagnosis of Down's syndrome entails tests such as amniocentesis which carry a presumed risk of causing miscarriage. No clear adverse effects of scans have been demonstrated (Ziskin, 1999), although they cannot be ruled out. Instructively, a large randomised UK trial involving 20000 women, was planned in the 1970s, but abandoned because the risks to be investigated were not clearly defined (Mole, 1986). But such vagueness itself arises from ignorance about low probability risks which can only be corrected by large-scale trials. Lack of evidence about risks can be elided into the assumption of safety. Screening scans also give rise to false negatives and positives, although very high positive predictive values can be achieved (Chitty *et al.*, 1991).

International and historical comparisons demonstrate that the difference in the organisational status of screening scans and prenatal genetic screening/testing cannot be attributed to their intrinsic features. The routinisation of universal prenatal screening for Down's syndrome has already taken place in the USA where, by the early 1990s, about two-thirds of women in antenatal care received serum screening

(Meaney, Riggle and Cunningham, 1993). In the UK, the uptake of serum screening increased from about one-third of the population of pregnant women in 1991, to about one-half in 1994, an increase which reflected both the greater availability and acceptance of the test (Wald *et al.*, 1996). A recent British Government report (Advisory Committee on Genetic Testing, 2000) recommended that prenatal genetic screening should be offered universally or to sub-populations collectively at low risk.

Press and Browner (1997) powerfully explain the creeping acceptance of novel, but problematic techniques such as serum screening in terms of the routinisation of medical innovation (McKinlay, 1982). The popular image of medicine as evidence-based practice implies that innovations are accepted only after rigorous cost-benefit analysis. However, McKinlay argued that the very introduction of large-scale feasibility studies creates an industry which then becomes self-sustaining. The enthusiasm with which the innovation is taken on board by those implementing it makes rejection by its intended beneficiaries less likely, because they accept the rational and altruistic claims of medicine at face value.

At the time of data collection, screening scans had been routinised at our hospital research site, whilst serum screening had not. However, several midwives suggested that the latter was beginning to become routine. No doctor offered such an insight. We may speculate that the marginal position, at our hospital research site, of midwives, who possess more knowledge than pregnant women, but are less involved in the genetic screening/testing process than hospital doctors, may have allowed them to detect routinisation processes not evident to these other two groups. However, the results of one survey (Fairgrieve *et al.*, 1997), which found that 87 per cent of a sample of midwives believed that prenatal screening for Down's syndrome should be offered to all women, suggests that many do not share the reservations discussed below.

The following, instructive quotation compares the anticipated routinisation of genetic screening with that already established for diagnostic scans.

Pregnant midwife: *I think they will eventually end up screening everybody because it is just the way. They will eventually get everybody to want one ... At one time a scan, you occasionally had a scan, and now everybody has a scan, along the board.* (Shirley, midwife, aged 34, interview, 20 weeks, no genetic tests)

A second midwife felt that a period of absence abroad had sensitised her to the recent change in status of genetic screening.

> **Pregnant midwife:** *I wasn't prepared to do that* [prenatal genetic screening/testing], *sort of, this whole new thing, because, before I went abroad, it was not so common to have these triple tests* [serum screening] *and things like that . . . And I remember being quite shocked when they, like, the midwives in* [neighbouring town] *were telling me . . . that they are offering all women these tests . . . Immediately I thought, 'Well, you're going to be doing really late terminations in some instances.' And I was really surprised by it all. But it never crossed my mind personally to have it* [genetic screening/testing] *done.* (Sharon, midwife, aged 31, interview, 36 weeks, no genetic tests)

Another midwife worried that an uninformed, consumer-driven adoption of new genetic screening/testing technology was taking place.

> **Midwife:** *It* [prenatal genetic screening/testing] *is becoming more and more commonplace, isn't it, and I think they are starting to accept it as part of the antenatal care. They seem to think that if they have got it in other areas, it is part of a service that perhaps they should be getting, so perhaps they should be having one so regardless of the implications. Because they haven't actually gone through it – 'Well, everybody else is having one, why shouldn't I have one? Is it just because you are trying to save money, the Health Service not providing a service?'* (Lane, midwife, interview)

We have already noted that consultants in our hospital would have liked to offer genetic screening/testing to all pregnant women, but were not prepared to do so unless a non-medical genetic counselling service was also funded. The neighbouring maternity hospital offered tests to all women, but with genetic advice provided by midwives.

Localised disparities, like those discussed in the above quotation, may trigger a technological levelling up process which contributes to routinisation. In the near future, genetic screening/testing may, as a result of such processes, acquire the same routine status at our hospital research site as screening scans. Those involved, pregnant women, doctors and midwives may then cease to regard their acceptance as requiring conscious choice.

The non-risk of stillbirths

Our present argument, that health-care systems focus selectively on, and define as risks, those contingencies which they deem problematically detectable and preventable will be further illustrated through a contrast between the degree of attention given to Down's syndrome, discussed above, with the almost total lack of concern which mothers expressed about stillbirths. The current starring risk status of Down's syndrome stands out both from the routine standing of spina bifida as a condition for which screening is required; and from the low profile of stillbirths, ignored at our hospital research site because screening was not considered possible.

Women at our hospital research site rarely worried about the risk of a stillbirth, as we shall see, even though, over the entire population, they faced a higher risk of experiencing a stillbirth than the abortion or birth of a baby with Down's syndrome. About 1 in 250 pregnancies of 24 or more weeks' gestation ends in a stillbirth (Gardosi *et al.*, 1998), whilst around 1 in 700 women will currently give birth to or abort a baby with Down's syndrome, as stated above. This discrepancy between relative probabilities and risk concern illustrates the power of socially organised selective attention.

The incidence of stillbirths has dropped substantially in the postwar period. Obstetricians have credited this reduction to advances in hospital procedures such as foetal heart monitoring (for example, Halliday *et al.*, 1995). However, this claim has been strongly contested, and it has been argued that the reduction may result from a more general improvement in the underlying health of the population (Tew, 1990, pp. 234–6). Increased risk of a stillbirth has been associated with both slow foetal growth and maternal smoking (Gardosi *et al.*, 1998).

Hospital doctors treated stillbirths as random in the sense that they believed that sub-populations of women at greater or lesser risk of this adverse event could not be identified in advance of a crisis. (One consultant at our hospital site linked this outcome to maternal smoking.) The following quotation, given by a pregnant midwife, conveys an almost frantic effort to identify risk markers for stillbirths, and so to meet one of the two conditions (the other being a means of prevention) required to make them preventable.

Pregnant midwife: *But before I went away, when I worked at the* [local hospital], *one of our consultants had a bit of a fixed idea about weight gain, and weight loss. And when we went to perinatal mortality* *meetings, I remember a few incidents of stillbirths where there had been a rapid weight loss very shortly beforehand, and was it indicative? We were always discussing this, and there's always two schools of thought with everything. And with this one, I think there must be four. And some would say, 'Oh it's a load of rubbish' . . . Obviously, there's been some more work done, and they've said it doesn't indicate anything . . . Having said that, if I suddenly lost a pound or so, I may become a bit more anxious. So I don't mind being weighed, at all, from that point of view.* (Sharon, midwife, aged 31, interview, 36 weeks, no genetic tests)

Despite rejecting the idea that maternal weight change could provide a stillbirth predictor, this pregnant midwife was concerned about the stability of her own weight. Her anxiety arose from second-order uncertainty, since weight variation had not been clearly eliminated as a risk marker.

All the women whom we interviewed, young and old, had thought about the risk of Down's syndrome. In contrast, stillbirths (as against miscarriages which were a common source of concern) were considered only by those who had previously encountered them, either through personal experience or, in the case of pregnant midwives, through their work. One woman became alarmed when she found out about the stillbirth of a baby born to another woman at the hospital. The following quotation illustrates the disturbing impact of direct experience of undiscussed risks.

Interviewer: *What kind of risks were you thinking of* [in relation to previous pregnancy].

Previously pregnant woman: *Well, I worried in case she was stillborn . . . I thought, 'Well, it's strange', I mean with it happening to* [sister], *'I'm going to be different than every other case.' But I thought, 'Our* [sister] *did everything the way she should, and she was unlucky' . . . And a few weeks before, a midwife had dropped a baby, at* [other hospital]. (Audrey, aged 39, post-partum, interview, serum screening)

This respondent put her sister's stillbirth down to the residual category of luck (Davison, Frankel and Davey Smith, 1992), and linked it to unpredictable accidents like dropping a baby. Her sense of vulnerability to chance contingencies may have been increased by exposure to an event for which neither cultural knowledge nor the maternity services would have prepared her.

Midwives knew about the risk of stillbirths through their professional experience.

Pregnant midwife: *I know people who have had stillbirths, and, you know, people are saying to me, 'Have you bought any equipment for the baby yet?'. And I say, 'Not yet'. And, I mean, I could almost see myself doing it into the last month, and rather reluctantly too, feeling like you are tempting fate . . . I think people are rather surprised. But in my midwifery training, I did encounter quite a number of stillbirths.* (Jackie, midwife, aged 36, interview, 14 weeks, no genetic tests)

This midwife held off from identifying with the baby because of fear of losing it through stillbirth, in the same way as did other women, not professionally acquainted with maternity care, who feared that a genetic abnormality might be identified (see Chapter 5). The latter could not worry about stillbirths because they did not recognise this risk. Midwives at the hospital with whom we have discussed this issue suggested that they did not want to alarm women about yet another contingency which could not be prevented. However, as a result of this protective reticence, women could not put personal experiences in a probabilistic context since the overall incidence of stillbirths had not been discussed with them. They could not counter the power of the availability heuristic by drawing upon the more complete, although still limited, probability heuristic.

2
Age and Pregnancy

Introduction

In this chapter, we will explore the diverse ways in which women understand the ageing process in relation to pregnancy and parenthood. We will use as a foil for this analysis social clock theory (Neugarten, Moore and Lowe, 1965; Neugarten, 1979, 1996), the idea that individuals make judgements about the timing of life transitions by calibrating them against temporal social norms.

Drawing primarily on the survey data, we will show that individual parental clocks tell different times. In order to explain this variability, we will introduce the concept of multiple biographical clocks, which we will illustrate with qualitative data. Women, individually and collectively, calibrate biographical time in numerous ways, generating different modes of ageing, for example chronological, historical, genetic, career and marital (see Table 2.4). An analytical framework based on the concept of multiple biographical clocks can be used to explore the impact of a historically novel timepiece, measuring maternal genetic age, on women's wider sense of themselves as early, late or on-time parents.

Social clock theory

Social clock theory provides an apparently simple, but powerful means of explaining and predicting a wide range of social behaviours. According to this theory:

> *There exists what might be called a prescriptive timetable for the ordering of major life events: a time in the life span when men and women are expected to marry, a time to raise children, a time to retire. This norma-*

tive pattern is adhered to, more or less consistently, by most persons in the society (Neugarten, Moore and Lowe, 1965, p. 711).

This theory asserts that societies delimit an approved age range for entry to, and exit from, socially defined roles. The lives of individuals will synchronise to a greater or lesser extent with such prescriptive timetables, and asynchrony will be negatively sanctioned. In this way, societies control the biographies of individuals, ensuring that activities essential to their maintenance, such as child-rearing, take place at the times in individuals' life cycles which are considered appropriate within the prevailing culture. Cultural differences in role timing, within the limits of the biologically possible, are well-documented. For example, in some African countries, girls are expected to marry and begin to bear children from the start of adolescence (Onolehemhen and Ekwempu, 1999). Reproduction at this age would be severely negatively sanctioned in many other societies. Social clocks prescribe idealised images of the timing of major life transitions, rather than merely statistical averages (Sorenson, 1995). Strictly speaking, therefore, social clock theory should only be applied to normative roles. But, in practice, the theory has been used to refine prediction of the effects on the individual of the whole range of positive and negative major life events, including, for instance, losing one's job or death of a spouse (Rook, Catalano and Dooley, 1989).

Neugarten, Moore and Lowe (1965) found, using survey data, that middle-class, adult Americans agreed quite closely about the best ages to undertake major role transitions, for example specifying optimum age ranges of about five years for getting married and becoming a grandparent. They also found that divergence between personal ideals and perceived norms declined with age during the adult period, and concluded that older adults, graduates of the school of hard knocks, become increasingly aware of the power of age discrimination. Neugarten (1979) proposed three social psychological forces which motivate individuals to stay on-time: firstly, social sanctions of approval and disapproval; secondly, the maintenance or loss of self-esteem through favourable or unfavourable comparisons with others; and, thirdly, the availability of social and instrumental support from peers within one's own age cohort.

Post-industrial societies may have become more fluid in their application of age norms (Neugarten and Neugarten, 1987). Some of our younger and older respondents justified their own chronological position by pointing to such a general loosening of age norms.

Interviewer: *How have you found people have reacted to your age?*
Pregnant midwife: *I think there's more and more women having them later and that.* (Gemma, aged 41, interview, 38 weeks, amniocentesis)
Interviewer: *Have you had anybody reacting not nicely because of your age, or anybody who has said anything?*
Pregnant woman: *No. I don't think it is that funny these days, now. Maybe, about 30 or 40 year ago it might have been. I think it has become more common for young girls to get pregnant now.* (Caroline, aged 18, interview, 20 weeks, no genetic tests)

Zepelin, Sills and Heath (1987) obtained partial support for the thesis that age norms have loosened in their replication of the study of temporal norms undertaken three decades earlier by Neugarten, Moore and Lowe (1965), summarised above. Comparisons of judgements made at these two time periods showed that the range of ages at which major role transitions were judged optimal had widened during this period, at least in the USA, suggesting that the prescriptive power of social clocks had weakened during the period following the Second World War. (Unfortunately for our present purpose, Zepelin, Sills and Heath could not compare judgements about the best age for having children as Neugarten, Moore and Lowe (1965) had not asked about this issue in their original study.) However, considerable consensus could still be observed in the 1980s in some areas, as reflected in low standard deviations for judged optimal ages for marriage, parenthood, finishing school and the start of a man's career. Hence, the timing of parenthood, according to this study, remains as one of a relatively small number of role transitions which, until the 1980s at least, was still influenced by a relatively consistent social clock. Its felt impact on both younger and older women is conveyed in the following two quotations.

Pregnant woman: *He* [husband] *kept putting it that it was our business, and it had nothing, well he's not that type of person normally. But he's kept saying, 'Oh, it's our business, got nothing to do with them* [work colleagues]'. *And I think he thought there would be a bit of stigma.* (Hilary, aged 40, interview, 23 weeks, amniocentesis)
Pregnant woman: *I did have some people who judged me and said, 'I will give you three weeks and the baby will be with* [foster] *parents'.*
Interviewer: *Who was that? What type of people was that?*
Pregnant woman: *Social workers and that.* (Caroline, aged 18, interview, 20 weeks, no genetic tests)

Social clock theory offers a significant advance over much more widely known psychological theories, which view human development as driven through a series of fixed, culturally universal stages by individuals' efforts to resolve internal contradictions inherent in each stage (Rossi, 1980). Such approaches can, in general, be criticised as culturally innocent (Douglas, 1994, p. 25), projecting the idiosyncrasies of middle-class, male, American culture within a particular historical period into universal of human nature. Featherman (1986) argued that, epistemologically, developmental stages can only be detected through the identification of aggregate commonalities in populations, and are therefore tied to the characteristics of particular historical cohorts. For example, Smelser and Halpern (1978) proposed that the emergence of developmental psychology in the early part of the twentieth century was associated with the establishment of age-rated school enrolment. Researchers who focus on cognitive changes within individuals can easily mistake institutional regularities for universal psychological stages of human development.

Social clock theory provides a valuable corrective to overly psychological analyses of the life course. But it suffers from a standard set of problems found in all approaches which attempt to explain human behaviour in terms of properties of an abstracted, reified social structure. The theory oversimplifies the complexities of normative judgements, leaving distinctions, for instance, between positively and negatively valued roles, and between role entry and exit, undifferentiated. Rook, Catalona and Dooley (1989) found that, with demographic variables such as social class, gender and ethnicity controlled for, the psychological impact of early versus late experience of life events depended upon how they were socially valued. Late timing of positive life events, including the birth of one's first child, was associated with psychological distress. However, late timing was more strongly related to mobilisation of social resources than to distress, suggesting that support and coping, rather than sanctions and punishment, are the predominant responses. But early occurrence of positive life events was not significantly related to either of these variables. Rook, Catalona and Dooley (1989) concluded that social clock theory is not empirically supported when positive and negative life events are differentiated, and demographic variables are controlled for.

We will argue below that present value judgements about the upper and lower age boundaries for parenting are based on complex, variable syntheses of beliefs about the nature of youth and middle age with medically inspired approaches to genetic risk prevention. Such judgements are not based on conventional rules, but on individual reasoning from broad, culturally mediated presuppositions, as argued, in relation to ageing, by Meyer (1986).

This process of concrete reasoning from broad principle is well-illustrated by cases, much discussed in the media, of women who, as a result of recent medical advances, have borne an implanted embryo well after the menopause. For example, Pauline Lyon gave birth to a second IVF baby at the age of 55, having lied about her age (51) when she had her first in order to cement a second marriage. Nevertheless, she was judged sympathetically. The clinic accepted her argument that '*it would be nice for her* [the first IVF child] *to have a little brother or sister*' (*Guardian*, 12/09/98). Mrs Lyon stated that '*I feel healthy enough to have one. I don't feel any different from when I had my first child.*' In relation to the future, she argued that, '*We know that we'll be 70 when the child is 15, but we're all living longer now.*' Her responses well illustrate the operation of a multiple biographical clock, relating, in this case, to parental age (the presence of a young sibling), marital age (a new marriage), vital age (good health) and lifespan age (a long life expectancy).

The meaning of the timing of parenthood depends upon the wider context in which it is located. This interpretive framework assumes that individuals generate contextualised temporal judgements in specific cases, drawing upon more abstract, culturally mediated principles. Similarities in judgements derive ultimately from shared cultural assumptions, for example about the 'natural' needs of young people or the impact of ageing on energy and fitness. We will now examine this issue through a detailed analysis of the opinions of one group of pregnant women.

The timing of parenthood

In this section, we will outline the main survey findings concerning pregnant women's views about the correct timing of parenthood, and discuss the relationships between these views and certain demographic variables. (Sampling and methods were summarised in the Methodology section of the Introduction.) This analysis will show, firstly, that, individually and collectively, our respondents' complex temporal judgements about parenthood cannot be explained in terms of the operation of a simple social clock; and, secondly, that attitudes to the timing of parenthood are associated with risk consciousness.

Age boundaries for parenthood

Survey data can document the complexity of judgements about the timing of parenthood, although it cannot bring out the reasoning behind such judgements with any depth. Our respondents were asked whether they felt that men and women could be too old or too young to have a baby, and, if so, to specify these age boundaries. Questions about age boundaries were asked in two stages in order to give respondents an explicit opportunity to decline to generate age judgements. As we shall see, the answers to these questions, taken together, show that our respondents, collectively, define the lower parental age boundary more sharply than the upper one, and are more accepting of older fatherhood than of older motherhood.

Answers to the four questions, which asked about the existence of upper and lower age limits, beyond which men and women should not become parents, are summarised in Figure 2.1 below.

Summary statistics describing the parenting age boundaries set by respondents who accepted such limits are presented in Table 2.1.

Figure 2.1 shows that pregnant women were more likely to identify age boundaries for younger than for older parents, and, at the older age, for women rather than men. Table 2.1 reveals greater variability in the age judgements which these women applied to older than to younger parents, with a closer consensus evident for women than for men

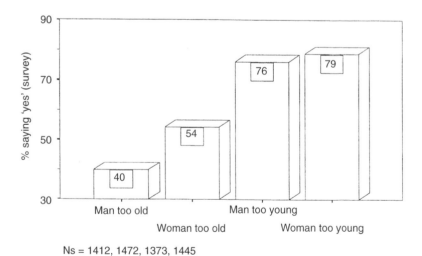

Figure 2.1 Can a Man or Woman be too Old or too Young to Have a Baby?

Table 2.1   The Appropriate Age Range for Parenting

	N	Mean (Year)	S.D. (Year)	Lowest age decile	Highest age decile
A woman too young?	1058	16.4	1.9	14	19
A man too young?	863	17.0	2.3	15	20
A woman too old?	772	42.8	5.0	37	50
A man too old?	494	48.7	7.2	40	60

Table 2.2   Correlations between the Ages at Which a Man and a Woman Are Judged too Old or Young to Have a Baby

Age relationship	Correlation	2-tailed significance	N
Man too young × woman too young	0.81	<0.001	841
Man too old × woman too old	0.50	<0.005	471
Woman too young × woman too old	−0.10	<0.01	679
Man too young × man too old	−0.10	<0.05	451

in each case. In short, our sample of pregnant women, collectively, operated a more widely and precisely defined normative social clock for early than for late entry into a parental role, and, to a lesser extent, for mothering than for fathering.

Analysis of relationships between an individual's age judgements attest to the complexity of the reasoning behind them. Some of the relationships between the ages at which a man or woman was judged too old or young to have a baby are summarised in Table 2.2 above.

As can be seen in Table 2.2, individual respondents judged the ages at which men and women would be too young to become parents more consistently than they did the ages at which they would be too old (correlations = 0.81 and 0.5 respectively). The statistically significant, but low, negative correlations between the ages at which a man or woman was judged too young and too old to become a parent, both −0.1, suggest a weak tendency for respondents who were more tolerant of older parenting to be more tolerant of younger parenting and vice versa. We can conclude, again, that the social clocks operated by our sample were more clearly defined at the lower than at the upper age boundary, and that individuals judge the age appropriateness of parenting in complex ways. Their age judgements were not regulated by a simple social clock.

Risk consciousness and attitudes to the timing of parenthood

Exploration of relationships between respondent characteristics and their endorsement of age limits for parenting can offer insights into why they were accepted or rejected. The analysis which follows will focus on comparisons of the 31 per cent of the sample who acknowledged all four age judgements (for older and younger fathers and mothers) with the 69 per cent who rejected at least one judgement by stating that men and/or women could not be too young and/or too old to become parents. Table 2.3 shows the results of a multivariate statistical analysis which related endorsement of parental age judgements to demographic variables by means of logistic regression. This analysis suggests that better-off women, and those who were concerned about the health of their baby, were more likely to endorse all four age judgements. A similar pattern to that displayed in Table 2.3, below, was found for each of the four individual age judgements. The meaning of the statistics presented in the Table is outlined below.

Socio-economic status was assessed by means of two questions, asking women whether they owned their own home and had a car in the household. Those who assented to both these questions were judged to have higher socio-economic status. (The results of this assessment matched quite closely with one based on conventional head of house-

Table 2.3 Predictors of Endorsement of Parental Age Norms (N = 1236)

Agree that men and women can be too young and too old to have a baby

Predictor	N	Odds (95% confidence intervals)	Probability
Socio-economic status			
lower	584	1	
higher	652	2.0 (1.5–2.5)	0.000
Concerned for health of baby			
no	1014	1	
yes	222	1.6 (1.1–3.2)	0.005

hold occupational status.) Older maternal age was also associated with endorsement of all four parental age judgements, but this variable dropped out of the analysis when socio-economic status was taken into account. The analysis shows that better-off women and those who answered 'yes' to a question asking if they had any concerns about the health of their baby were more likely to endorse all four parental age norms.

The odds ratios given in Table 2.3 and other Tables provide estimates of the relative chances of the event in question occurring within the sub-groups indicated. For example, the first part of the Table shows that better-off women were twice as likely as poorer women to endorse all four age norms (relative odds = 2.0). The computed odds allow for relationships with other variables which were included in the final, most accurately predictive model. In this case, the relationships observed cannot be explained in terms of associations with maternal age, marital status, parity or history of previous pregnancy problems. The 95 per cent confidence levels provide a measure of the accuracy of the estimated odds. There is a 95 per cent probability, for example, that the just mentioned odds ratio in the population from which the sample is drawn lies between 1.5 and 2.5.

The statistical interaction between socio-economic status and concern for the health of the baby was statistically insignificant, and was eliminated from the model. A statistical interaction occurs when the relationship between two variables is itself associated with the values of other variables. For example, if it had been found that better-off women were more likely to endorse all four parental age norms only if they were concerned about the health of their baby, then it could be said that a woman's probability of being tested was affected by the interaction of socio-economic status and health concern. However, no evidence of this or other statistical interactions was obtained.

Conclusions derived from multivariate, cross-sectional analysis must always be treated with caution, for two reasons. Firstly, only weakly predictive aggregate relationships can be expected when complex, multi-determined processes involving feedback are analysed. Nevertheless, these relationships can provide clues about underlying social processes. Secondly, explanatory models induced from multivariate analysis are affected by the selection of variables for entry into the predictive equation. Although the researcher can try out different combinations of variables, so as to test out the stability of the model which emerges in the final regression equation, it is not possible to explore the effects of variables which were not incorporated into the research design. Hence, only tentative claims can be made about the empirical grounding of the emergent model, which might require revision if new predictor variables were introduced. Because of these limitations, nomothetic statistical analysis can usefully be complemented by a qualitative exploration of the social process in question.

We can only speculate as to the explanation of the relationships summarised in Table 2.3. The association between socio-economic status and greater use of age judgements for parenting may reflect a broader tendency for more prosperous people to seek greater control of their social and physical environment, perhaps because they can afford to pay more for the luxury of risk avoidance (Lefcourt, 1992; Heyman and Huckle, 1993).

Similarly, the relationship between concern for the health of the baby and the tendency to make judgements about parental age may arise because health anxiety forms an element in a more general risk aversion. A comparable, independent but statistically insignificant, trend was found for women who were concerned about their own health to be more likely to endorse all four age judgements. Individuals who worry about health may also seek to avoid risks which they link to parenting outside the culturally normal age range. All of the above effects were obtained with maternal age statistically controlled for.

As will be seen in Chapter 4, women with health concerns, and those of higher socio-economic status, were also more likely to be offered genetic tests. We will argue that this relationship may occur because doctors responded to women's anxiety by offering them genetic tests. Risk consciousness, and the higher socio-economic status to which it was related, were associated both with timekeeping about parenthood and the processing of women through the genetic risk management system.

Dimensions of parental age

The above survey data offers only a limited overview of pregnant women's parental age judgements. To learn more, we need to consider the ways in which individuals make sense of their world, drawing upon wider cultural belief systems which they mark with their own individual stamp. The analysis which follows will be based mainly on qualitative interview data, although we will also consider the reasons which women gave for their survey responses. We will be concerned primarily with reasoning about the upper age barrier, the main focus of this book in relation to prenatal genetic screening/testing. But we will also consider, by way of comparison, respondents' explanations of why they thought that a man or woman could be too young to become a parent.

We will show that women's thinking about maternal age drew upon a highly complex, multidimensional set of time calibrations, outlined in Table 2.4, below, which generated a set of variable age categorisations and value judgements.

The maternal genetic clock which medical advance has recently introduced coexists with the other biographical clocks listed in Table 2.4, all telling separate times.

A pregnant woman could be 'young' in some respects, but 'old' in others. The complexity of the chronological calculations which respondents performed can easily be overlooked because the underlying constructs of time are embedded implicitly in their reasoning about what is to count as 'too old' or 'too young'. Moreover, such reasoning tends to be taken for granted within Western cultures in which the evaluation of time usage plays such a central role.

Although these age dimensions are all more or less loosely associated with chronological ageing, women saw themselves as growing older in different ways at varying rates. For example, a respondent might rebut the implicit accusation that she had started parenthood too late by arguing that her vitality had not diminished as she grew older; or explain later parenting in terms of its timing in relation to a marriage which took place relatively late in life. Lippman (1999) has developed

Table 2.4 Dimensions of Parental Age

Parental age dimension	**Parental age referent**
Birth	Age when a particular child is born
Parenthood	Age when first child is born
Vital	Age-related energy and fitness
Lifespan	Future life expectancy
Project	Timing of parenthood project
Apparent	Appearance of ageing
Historical	Psycho-social distance from other age cohorts
Other role	e.g. time married, career point
Genetic	Age-related risk of foetal genetic abnormalities
Medical	Age-related risk of all medical complications

a similar analysis with respect to the *'embodied'* way that older pregnant women assess their age in relation to personal circumstances, of which genetic risk comprises just one component.

The ten age dimensions set out in Table 2.4, and their use in value judgements about parental age, will now be considered with respect to our qualitative, and, in one instance, quantitative research data.

Birth age

Birth age refers simply to the age of the parents at the time a particular child is born. Our interview respondents rarely made absolute value judgements about raw, biological age which, unusually, is referenced directly in the following quotation.

> **Interviewer:** *What age do you think of as being older?*
> **Pregnant woman:** *Em, fifties. You see some old mum taking their children to school who's in their fifties. And I think that looks old, like for a little un, you know what I mean? It's not old, but . . .* (Maureen, aged 18, interview, 20 weeks, no genetic tests)

By distancing herself from older parenting, this respondent perhaps sought to strengthen the legitimacy of her own position as a relatively young mother. She conveys a sense of the intrinsic wrongness, for her, of a woman in her fifties looking after a young child. However, her qualification that, in some other sense, a person in their fifties is *'not old'* illustrates this young woman's multidimensional understanding of age. In an era of increased life expectancy, an individual may be judged old as a parent, but not old as a person. This historically recent increase in life expectancy has uncoupled parental from personal ageing.

Some older respondents resented being subjected to critical judgements based on unthinking assumptions about the proper age for parenting. The respondent quoted below rejected this absolutist view, and had changed her GP because he had attempted to impose his own arbitrary age judgements upon her.

> **Pregnant woman:** *I think it's more my age. I seem to get it from all quarters. Before I planned on having another baby, I seen the GP for the contraceptive pill. And I think I was only 33, so [son] was still only a baby really. And he says, 'A woman of your age should not be taking this. Have you not thought about being sterilised?'. So really, ever since then, I've*

> *thought, 'God, I'm over the hill here'. But, luckily the GP, it's a group prac-*
> *tice, and I've chosen the only lady doctor on the practice. And I've chosen*
> *the doctor I wanted, and she's really good. She's never said anything about*
> *my age. If I've asked her questions, she's answered it as honestly as she*
> *could, which, at the end of the day, that's all you want.* (Diane, aged 38,
> interview, 16 weeks, no genetic tests)

The male GP was resented and rejected because he had, according to this respondent's account, attempted to impose an 'undelimited' approach to expertise (Heyman and Henriksen, 1998a, pp. 56–8) predicated on his own unexamined assumptions about parental age. The respondent sought a 'liberal' approach to expertise, with facts separated from values, and the expert supplying only the former. Social clock theory, discussed above, maintains that parental and other age norms are sustained through the sanction of disapproval. But, as the last quotation demonstrates, social actors do not passively accept surface judgements about parental age limits, but question the assumptions which underlie them.

Parenthood age

A person's age as a parent can be distinguished from their age at the birth of a particular child simply because, for those who have more than one child, this event can occur at different points in their parenting career. Attitudes towards birth age may be affected by its location in the chronology of parenthood, as illustrated by the following quotation.

> **Pregnant woman:** *That's when we really started trying* [to have a baby], *like, that's when I hit 25. I was thinking, I could be, like, by the time I go into this fertility clinic, and by the time something happens I could be 28, 29, and only have one. What happens if I want more and the age starts, like?* (Samantha, aged 25, interview, no genetic testing)

This respondent projected forward her age at the birth of subsequent children into her thirties, an age which she defined as unacceptably old. This calculation, in turn, made an age of 28 or 29 too late for the birth of her first child. The notion that *'the age starts'* suggests that this respondent saw herself as drifting towards a temporal boundary beyond which parenthood would become problematic.

The woman quoted below assessed herself as maternally old and medically at risk at the age of 35 because she was expecting her first child.

> **Pregnant woman:** *I mean, being 35, I think that's quite old to have your first one really. I mean we got married when we were 33, so we are having a family later on in life. But I mean, as I say, everything is alright up to now, hopefully.* (Maria, aged 36, interview after taped hospital consultation [Bell], 15 weeks, serum screening)

She explained her older parenthood age in terms of her younger marital age (see *'Age and Non-Parental Roles'*, below).

The older respondent quoted below felt that she had been stigmatised more at the birth of her first child, even though she was older when she gave birth to her subsequent children.

> **Pregnant woman:** *I must say, I had a worse reaction to my age with my first baby. And that was really, you know, 'How old are you, how old?' and, 'This is your first, your first'. And I was thinking, 'I'm not old', you know what I mean? I was only 33, you know, it was around about 34, and then the other one around 36, and this one around about 38.* (Doreen, aged 38, interview, 28 weeks, no genetic tests)

If a woman makes a relatively late start to her parenting career, in her early 30s, then she might not have her last child until she is over 40. This respondent, perhaps, redeemed herself, in relation to the parental clock operated by others, by giving birth to three children in a relatively short space of time, thus catching up with their temporal timetable. Like the first woman quoted in this section, she struggled to make sense of multiple ageing velocities, asserting that she was *'not old'* at 33, in a general sense, even though treated as old with respect to becoming a first-time parent. However, she set the boundary for being an old parent at a considerably later age than did the first, younger respondent cited.

Vital age

Although average energy levels may decline with increasing age, individual trajectories vary considerably, depending upon a person's mental and physical health, fitness and lifestyle. Hence, vital and chronological age could be more or less uncoupled, depending upon how their relationship was conceptualised. Younger women sometimes expressed gloomy views about the ageing trajectory, suggesting that older parents would be too decrepit to cope with looking after children.

> **Pregnant woman:** *I want to be young enough to think that I'm fit enough to enjoy them while I'm young, but I don't think the fact of being older as a risk to the baby entered me head.* (Sheila, aged 25, interview, 24 weeks, no genetic tests)

This last quotation directly juxtaposes wider social with medical concerns, which the respondent ruled out as a consideration influencing her preference for younger parenting. This wider concern could, itself, be contextualised, as the energy required of parents depends upon the social circumstances in which they bring up children.

> **Pregnant woman:** *And this is an issue that looms in my head a lot. They* [respondent's parents] *had no money, and they were always tired. And I just don't feel that we got the attention that we needed, because I think they were just too tired, because they were older and they couldn't buy in help.* (Jackie, midwife, aged 36, interview, 14 weeks, no genetic tests)

This respondent saw the damaging effects of age on parenting capacity as mediated by socio-economic circumstances, with the reduction in energy which she equated with ageing compounded by poverty. Parenting, on this view, demands less of those who, like the Royal Family, can uphold family values with the help of nannies, tutors and servants. By implication, the presumed damaging effects of age on vitality could be mitigated through the use of material resources, and involved more than a purely biological process.

Respondents who accepted a link between parental ageing and decline in vitality could plot the slope of the implicit graph linking these two variables differently. Women in their 20s, like the woman of 25 quoted above, tended to locate the start of this anticipated decline in the 30s, whilst women in their 30s often pushed it back beyond their own age.

> **Pregnant woman:** *If I hadn't got pregnant, sort of, by the time I was 38, then we had seriously considered that we wouldn't have any more ... I mean, it was me age, because I think the older you get, it's got to be slightly harder for you, and also for the children as well, you know, when they get older, and they have older parents. And also, you haven't got that*

energy, I don't think, to contribute. (Tracy, aged 38, interview, 29 weeks, serum screening)

The age boundary of 38 which she set as the acceptable upper limit for having a baby would have been regarded as too old by many younger women.

The next quotation illustrates the complexity of judgements about vitality. These could encompass physical and mental energy, and be affected by negotiations with significant others.

Pregnant woman: *I really did think I was too old to even go in for another one, not physically, just, em, mentally . . . And* [husband] *has always, big* [husband] *has always been, 'You're not old, come on, we could have'. And* [husband] *would, he would have lots of kids. So, that side to it has always been him making me feel that I'm not too old, but me still contradicting it. And when you're throwing up and everything, it's like, 'I told you I was too old'. And he's rubbing me back.* (Lesley, aged 37, interview, 26 weeks, amniocentesis)

The support which this woman received from her husband, and his insistence that she was *'not old'* appear to have persuaded her to overcome the mental burn-out which, otherwise, might have prevented her from having further children.

Other women challenged, in various ways, the package which linked ageing, energy decline and ability to parent. The next respondent quoted believed that she could draw upon her own coping resources to offset this presumed decline.

Pregnant woman: *But I'm classed as what you call 'mature mother', so people say, and 'Good grief! How are you going to cope? You must be mad, having children at your age' . . . But most people know me very well, and they know I will cope. My best friend next door, she says, 'Oh, you will cope, I know you'll cope', 'cos I do cope with most things.* (Patricia, aged 37, interview, 24 weeks, serum screening)

By asserting her ability to cope with the effects of ageing, the above respondent implicitly accepted the trajectory of diminishing vitality. This assertion legitimated her position as a pregnant woman of 37, and thus overrode the social clock based on the assumption of an inevitable vitality decline during middle age. But the price paid for this rebuttal is heightened individualisation of responsibility (Beck-Gernsheim, 1996).

This woman took personal responsibility for managing parenthood despite the presumed burden of age. Another respondent related her own ability to cope to the quality of support received from her partner.

> **Pregnant woman:** *I just react when, I, like, em, I'm going to be 60 when the baby will be 20 . . .*
> **Interviewer:** *Does that concern you?*
> **Pregnant woman:** *No, not, em, with the partner I've got, because with my son and daughter, well, with the daughter actually, the son's been no bother, with my daughter, I've had nobody . . . But this time I will. That doesn't bother us.* (Gemma, aged 41, interview, 38 weeks, amniocentesis)

The ability of individuals to cope with a particular demand depends upon the interpersonal and material support available, as well as on their individual capabilities. By drawing upon these wider sources of support, women could share a responsibility which, in contemporary Western societies, still tends to fall ultimately on them. The perceived availability of high-quality social support enabled the woman quoted to maintain temporal legitimacy even though she was giving birth towards the end of her child-bearing period.

The last two responses were based on an implicit developmental theory which assumes that ageing entails an unavoidable decline in energy. The women quoted avoided placing themselves on the wrong side of an age boundary for parenting by uncoupling personal and family coping from levels of vitality. Other older respondents questioned this developmental theory.

> **Pregnant woman:** *I had one at 26, our* [daughter] *is nine, and this one I don't feel any different really. I feel I'm more able to cope. I know it sounds ridiculous, but, even when I was 26, I thought I was able to cope. So I don't know it is different. We are older now, but I don't feel any different from when I had our* [daughter]. (Shirley, midwife, aged 34, interview, 20 weeks, no genetic tests)

This respondent bracketed her feeling that age had not made a difference as apparently *'ridiculous'*, that is, as implausible to others, but true, nevertheless. She saw her own experience that, if anything, she could cope better when older as contradicting the received wisdom which equates age with declining energy.

Those who challenged this equation could only do so by drawing on their own experience. Hence, their challenges were confined to the present, pitting personal experience against accepted, but not necessarily personally valid, generalisations about ageing trajectories. This confinement to the present is articulated in the next quotation.

Interviewer: *How have you found your age with the pregnancy?*
Previously pregnant midwife: *No problem at all apart from that* [genetic] *test, really. I would say I felt healthier and had more energy this time, which I was surprised at, then.* (Jessica, midwife, aged 42, interview, post-partum, amniocentesis)

Just as the previously quoted respondent expected her experience of an absence of age-related change to appear ridiculous, so this woman felt *'surprised'* that she had enjoyed greater vitality during her current pregnancy than during earlier ones. The question raised about this positive experience suggests its anomalous status relative to culturally shared assumptions about the relationship between age and energy.

As well as uncoupling the decline associated with ageing from ability to cope, and questioning the association itself, older women could justify the timing of their pregnancies by balancing the presumed drawbacks of later parenting against its advantages, particularly increased maturity and possession of a greater wealth of experience.

Previously pregnant midwife: *Oh yes, I think there are advantages in being an older parent. There are obvious disadvantages, but I think there are advantages. We've got maturity to offer them, and I think that we have had the opportunity to do the things that you want to do in your own right. In some ways, it's probably more difficult in that respect, being an older parent in terms of . . . you know what the freedom is like. You know more of what you are missing in a way sometimes. On the other hand, you've got a lot to offer the children.* (Jessica, midwife, aged 42, interview, post-partum, amniocentesis)

This point was rarely appreciated by doctors and midwives who had learnt to view older maternity as primarily a risk.

Age in relation to the life span

Future life expectancy, like vitality, may be expected to decline as a result of the ageing process, but varying assumptions can be made about its rate. Parents who have children take on an obligation which can last for more than 20 years. Their projected ability to meet this obligation depends upon their anticipated longevity as well as their expectation of future health at the time a child is born. The following, youthful respondent expressed a pessimistic view of the years of life remaining to middle-aged people. She used this view to justify rejection of older parenting.

> **Interviewer:** *What do you think about the older women who are having babies?*
> **Pregnant woman:** *Oh I think they are, I've got nowt against them, but I think like, I don't think you should be too old.*
> **Interviewer:** *As in what?*
> **Pregnant woman:** *Like 40 and all that, because really they are not going to live . . . Say I had a bairn at 40, I wouldn't want that bairn to grow up and be about 10, and then, at 50, I'd have a heart attack, and I would die, see. So, no, it's no age to have a bairn, then, like.* (Fiona, aged 18, interview, 24 weeks, no genetic tests)

The youngest mothers may emphasise disadvantages of older parenting, such as heightened risk of genetic abnormalities and limited longevity, in order to defend their own temporal position against accusations of irresponsibility. The woman quoted had just explained that she did not want to attend parenting classes, and did not go out very much, because she feared that other people would call her *'a slag'* for becoming pregnant so young. Her statement about having *'got nowt against'* older mothers, as well as her exaggerated representation of mortality rates among women aged 50, can be understood in relation to the stigmatisation of the chronology of her own parenthood, as well as to the negative view of age found in a youth-oriented culture.

Older women also expressed concern that if they gave birth in their mid-30s, they would be drawing towards the end of their lifespan by the time the child had grown up, and would face increased risk that the parental project would be disrupted by health problems. The woman quoted below gave this as one of her reasons for not wanting children after the age of about 36. (Her pregnancy had been unplanned.)

> **Previously pregnant midwife:** *And, I suppose, not being able to do as much with them, being old parents. When they are in their teens, we will be near retiring.* (Jessica, midwife, aged 42, interview, post-partum, amniocentesis)

This concern extended to grandparents who could not cope with the demands of young children in extreme old age.

> **Previously pregnant midwife:** *But I think one of the disadvantages of being older, also, is the children miss out having a lot to do with their grandparents. I mean, my parents, my father is 80, and my mother is 75, and they are limited in what they can do. They are limited in their tolerance, yes.* (Jessica, midwife, aged 42, interview, post-partum, amniocentesis)

Children born to older parents would have to cope both with elderly grandparents during their childhood, and with parents ready to retire during their young adulthood.

Older women could rebut these arguments, and legitimate their pregnancy timing, by arguing that, in modern conditions, the ageing process has been significantly slowed down.

> **Pregnant woman:** *It just depends on the individual, doesn't it, 'cos, you see, some ladies at 40 and 50, and they've got lovely figures. I would say, maybe, 50 is getting a bit too old, like, but the 40s, I think that's great, 'cos it's a different lifestyle nowadays.* (Wendy, aged 35, interview, 29 weeks, serum screening)

If ageing is linked to lifestyle, rather than merely the passage of time, then people can vary their life expectancy. This argument weakens the legitimacy of the parental social clock as a general regulatory device.

The timing of the parental project

Respondents often treated parenthood as a project which would absorb much of their time and energy for a substantial but limited period of their lives, during which directly personal goals would be set aside. By bounding parenthood with periods of childlessness, couples could balance self-expression against the other-centred activity of procreation. (For the sake of simplicity, we will use the term 'end' of parenthood to refer to a trajectory of declining responsibility, which is normally associated with young adulthood, but which may vary if, for example, a child has a learning disability, cannot obtain employment, or requires support as a single parent.) These free periods were seen as enabling parents-to-be to charge their batteries before embarking on parenthood, and to recover afterwards. As will be seen, at the end of this chapter (see Figure 2.2, p. 94), the notion of project timing was applied more frequently to the beginning than to the end of parenthood, but was discussed in relation to each. Commonly, older women saw young adulthood as a time for self-fulfilment which would be wasted through becoming a parent too early.

> *There is so much to do when you are young, and plenty of time later for children.* (Questionnaire)

The following young pregnant woman expressed a similar view.

> **Pregnant woman:** *Nah, nah, it's too young. I mean I've wasted, I mean my life's gone now, with us being pregnant. And, I mean, I'm going to have a baby in January, and then I'm going to be 19 in September. And my whole life's just, I mean I've got to bring a baby up and everything. It's just going to be my whole life, and I haven't enjoyed myself yet. So I'm not regretting it, but, ehm, like, I disagree with me age, with me being so young.* (Fiona, aged 18, interview, 24 weeks, no genetic tests)

This respondent's sense of loss at not having *'enjoyed myself yet'* was based on two implicit assumptions: that this period of self-expression needed to take place before the exhausting project of parenthood was embarked upon; and that parenthood precluded personal fulfilment.

Additionally, older respondents were concerned that young girls should not miss out on their education on account of becoming pregnant too young.

> *Need qualifications first.* (Questionnaire)
> *As long as they have finished their education.* (Questionnaire)

Younger pregnant women did not necessarily feel, however, that they were missing out. The widespread view of youth as essentially a time for learning and enjoyment belongs to a culturally derived belief system about the development of human nature. The following young respondent commented on her surprise at discovering that she did not mind the restriction of opportunities for socialising which resulted from her pregnancy.

Interviewer: *Are you finding that you're going out less now?*
Pregnant woman: *Don't know.* [I] *used to be out every single week-end. During the week. And since I've found out I'm pregnant, I've been out twice. It hasn't bothered us . . . Everyone else was going clubbing – 'See you later!'.*
Interviewer: *How does that make you feel?*
Pregnant woman: *It doesn't bother us, which I'm pleased about. I thought it would have, but it hasn't.* (Maureen, aged 18, interview, 20 weeks, no genetic tests)

Just as some older women discovered, to their surprise, that their energy had not declined, so, this young woman experienced disconfirmation of her expectation, derived from the standard model of young adult human nature, that she would suffer from enjoyment deprivation. She also challenged the view that parenthood necessarily entailed the complete abandonment of other social roles and contacts.

Interviewer: *Were your parents, or were you, concerned at all about your age?*
Pregnant woman: *No, 'cos I know peoples who is younger than me who's had them. They've managed fine. 'Cos I know, like, after I'd told her* [mother], *I knew that, when she'd calmed down, she would be alright, and she was. And she was saying, em, when I've had it, at least twice a week she'll be taking the baby off us, so I can go out, so I'm not stuck in the house with the baby.* (Maureen, aged 18, interview, 20 weeks, no genetic tests)

The above respondent used social comparisons with mothers younger than herself who had managed successfully as evidence supporting her case that she could cope with the parenting project. Such comparisons are more readily available in areas, including the one in which the present research was undertaken, which have high teenage pregnancy rates. If one of the main principles underlying the operation of social clocks for the start of parenting is that very young parents miss out on other life experiences, and if the extent to which they are deprived depends upon the degree of social support available, then the settings on this clock should take account of a young parent's social network. Absolute temporal judgements dissolve when the meaning of the chronology of parenthood is considered in individual cases. Similarly, the absence of desired social support could exacerbate the restriction of opportunities to explore other roles resulting from early entry into parenthood.

Pregnant woman: *He* [father] *is expecting me to look after him, feed him, bring up this baby by myself. He is not going to do anything to help me. And I said, 'You have got to be fair. Look at it from my point of view. I have given up my life once for one baby' . . . All I want is his help. I am not asking him to marry me and tie him down with six kids.* (Caroline, aged 18, interview, 20 weeks, no genetic tests)

Such a lack of support, in effect, made young women younger in relation to the parenting project because it made the required sacrifice of other role opportunities more severe.

Although many of our older respondents saw the need for self-centred enjoyment as an essential characteristic of young adult human nature, younger women assessed their own needs in relation to their lifestyles, and to the reference groups with whom they identified. The next respondent quoted identified with the older women with whom she shared factory work, and so did not *'feel young'*.

Interviewer: *Did your age worry you, that you were pregnant so young? Do you not feel that you are so young?*
Pregnant woman: *I don't feel young because, in the factory, they are all older than me, and I am the youngest in the factory, but I don't feel young.* (Donna, aged 17, interview, 20 weeks, no genetic tests)

This respondent defined her own age in terms of that of the group with whom she identified, an entirely reasonable procedure if the timing of the parenting project is judged in relation to its impact on a person's wider life.

If the timing of parenthood is thought about in terms of the commencement and termination of a project, then an early start enables the project to be finished more quickly, allowing more time for other forms of self-fulfilment later in life, as several younger pregnant women pointed out.

Pregnant woman: *Me mam said, 'It will grow up with you. And, like, when you are, like, 20, and the bairn will be about five, you'll be able to, like, still go out and do what you want to do.'* (Alice, aged 14, interview, 24 weeks, no genetic tests)

Hence, a condition which current government policy defines as problematic could appear both culturally normal and beneficial to women brought up in localities with a tradition of teenage pregnancies (Aarvold and Buswell, 1999).

The reader may be thinking that such responses involve defensive rationalisation of an unfortunate position. Similarly, the experience of the young woman, quoted above, who was surprised to discover that she couldn't be *'bothered'* to go out might be explained in terms of the hormonal and physical changes associated with pregnancy. However, this explaining away of young pregnant women's perspectives in terms of their putative causes rests on an implicit assumption about human development: that young adults need to go through a period of individualistic self-expression. Causal explanation of beliefs about oneself or the world come onto the agenda only when their rationality has been explicitly, or, more usually, implicitly rejected.

Just as some very young mothers regretted the loss of opportunities to enjoy other activities which, they felt, their early pregnancy entailed, so, some older respondents accounted for delayed parenthood in terms of their wish to enjoy more hedonistic activities to the full whilst still young.

Interviewer: *Why had you not wanted to have a family* [earlier]*?*
Previously pregnant midwife: *Because we were too selfish, and enjoying our holidays and lifestyle, two cars, and you name it, not having to be tied. We just couldn't see ourselves as parents.* (Tina, midwife, aged 37, interview, post-partum, serum screening)

The contrast, implied in this quotation, between the selfish nature of married childlessness and the selflessness of parenthood underpinned much of the discussion of the timing of the parental project. Selfishness, in this sense, appears to be culturally licensed during young adulthood, but its eventual abandonment is required. This respondent's mild self-reproof was probably associated with her view of herself as having dallied too long before taking the plunge into parenthood. However, as we have already noted, this underlying contrast could be challenged by those who argued that young adults were not naturally selfish in this sense.

We have seen that the youngest pregnant women could legitimate their timing of the parental project by pointing to the temporal space which they would enjoy at its end. Similarly, later parenting could be criticised for squeezing out this space. One respondent had set a personal age limit of 38 for becoming pregnant on various grounds, one of which was that becoming a parent after this age *'doesn't give you any more time in your twilight years'* (Tracy, aged 38, interview, 29 weeks, serum screening). The next respondent discussed her mother's feeling that she had missed out on a period of privacy with her husband at the end of the parental project as a result of a late pregnancy.

> **Pregnant woman:** *It's like my mum, she had a baby when she was 42, my mum. So I have a sister, 13, and my mum says she wouldn't part with her or anything. She loves her to bits, but she says, 'I've been having kids since I was 19 year old, and now it's time me and your dad were having time on our own'. And I think she wants something a bit better for us, you know – 'Don't have any too late because you need time on your own, when you get a little bit older'. See, they're in their 50s now, and [mother's daughter]'s still at school.* (Patricia, aged 37, interview, 24 weeks, serum screening)

Parenting, on this view, needs to be buffered, at both its beginning and end, by extended holidays which allow time for more self-expressive activities. This culturally mediated perspective assumes both that individuals naturally need such holidays, and that parenthood is, essentially, a time of altruistic sacrifice.

Apparent ageing

As with vitality and lifespan, the appearance of ageing may be more or less uncoupled from birth age. A person may look younger or older than expected in relation to what is considered normal within a specific historical period, either within a particular socio-economic group, or within the wider society. The quotation given at the beginning of the book, from a novel set in eighteenth-century Paris, well illustrates the dramatic shifts in expectations about ageing which have occurred, and continue to occur, over a relatively short historical time period.

Responses which parents receive, or anticipate, from others may depend upon how old they look, or believe themselves to look.

> **Pregnant woman:** *I've never been one of these that looks young, so, sometimes, people think I look older than what I am. And people's looking at me, and he [husband] says, 'You're imagining it', and I say, 'I'm not.' I felt as if everybody's looking at us at the Metro.* (Lesley, aged 37, interview, 26 weeks, amniocentesis)

This woman's painful self-consciousness concerning others' temporal judgements about her pregnant status was underpinned by a double presumption: that they would see her as older than her chronological age; and that her apparent age would make her stand out as an object of censorious attention. Hence, she suffered for appearing to violate a norm generated by the parental social clock. Her husband's attempted reassurance seems, in this case, to have failed.

A woman's apparent age could create uncertainty about her parental status. Experience of the resulting embarrassment motivated the respondent quoted below to avoid becoming, according to her own calibration, an 'old mother'.

> **Pregnant woman:** *I don't want to be an old mother because I have a memory of a friend of mine, a school mate of mine. And her parents were so old that, when she went for walks with them, people would sometimes ask her if she was going for a walk with her grandparents, and made her feel very uneasy and awkward.* (Kate, aged 32, interview, 20 weeks, no genetic tests)

Equivocal situations, which can equally well be defined in one of two distinct ways (Harré and Secord, 1972) cause intense social disruption, and even farce, because social actors do not know which interpretive/normative framework they should draw upon in order to understand the meaning of socially situated actions. Moreover, attempts at clarifying the definition of the situation, such as asking the child whether she was being accompanied by her parents or grandparents, create further social embarrassment by drawing attention to the perceived normative lapse which gave rise to the initial equivocation.

One older mother had directly experienced this equivocal situation, and had noticed that others attempted to clarify it covertly.

> **Interviewer:** *Did you ever have any responses to your age, with you being pregnant, from anybody?*
> **Previously pregnant midwife:** *Not really overt responses. Things like, I mean, this happens fairly often I suppose, people don't quite know whether to call you the child's mother or not . . . You know, they will say to the children something, 'Is that your mother or your grandmother?'.* (Jessica, midwife, aged 42, interview, post-partum, amniocentesis)

Inevitably, consideration of apparent age raised questions of gender politics.

Previously pregnant midwife: *And there is a child at the moment at school who asked me if I was* [child's] *mam, things like that.*
Interviewer: *How do you react to that?*
Previously pregnant midwife: . . . *It bothers me in terms of whether it will affect them, but it doesn't really, it doesn't bother me. And it's funny because* [husband] *doesn't get that.* (Jessica, midwife, aged 42, interview post-partum, amniocentesis)

The survey data, discussed above, showed that pregnant women themselves define parental age limits more tightly for women than for men. However, older mothers attempted to legitimate their positions. The above respondent gently challenged the implicit social clock, against which she had been judged tardy, by pointing out gender inequalities in its operation. Clocks which keep inconsistent times, she implies, cannot be trusted.

In relation to her own children, the above respondent had not just passively accepted her maternal age as problematic, but had entered into negotiations with her young son about its acceptability.

Previously pregnant midwife: *I, I feel embarrassed when people say to me, from the point of view of the children's hearing, you know, whether they will be affected by it. But I mean, I've talked to* [child] *about it, whether it bothers him. He said no.* (Jessica, midwife, aged 42, interview, post-partum, amniocentesis)

The following two quotations represent the social impact of the gap between apparent and birth age as black comedy.

Pregnant woman: *When I, we went to the clinic the first time, . . . I was making a joke of it . . . I says, 'I'll put me make-up on, do me hair'. And, of course, I gets booked in, you know, and she* [midwife] *went, 'And how old are you* [first name]*? And I went, 'I'm 40'. So she writes 40, then she underlines it in red three times. The effort I'd made to put meself right. And it was lovely, because it was very quiet, and there was only a couple of more girls in before me. And I was quite relieved, tell you the truth . . . 'Cos I was saying, ee, if I was, I would be very self-conscious, you know.* (Hilary, aged 40, interview, 23 weeks, amniocentesis)

This woman, according to her own account, had dressed herself up in an attempt to look younger, but her efforts had been subverted by the action of the admitting midwife who had highlighted her as a high-risk case. Although this respondent presented her predicament as a farce, it clearly had a serious side, causing her to feel *'self-conscious'*, and, perhaps, reducing her willingness to attend subsequent clinic appointments.

The woman quoted below described an equivocal situation in which she was, at first, mistakenly classified as a younger, and so not medically problematic, pregnant woman.

Pregnant woman: *I was just getting out when this nurse came up to the counter, and she said, 'Has Mrs* [surname] *gone?'. And I said, 'No, I'm Mrs* [surname]. *And she said, 'No' – this is a nice midwife – and she said, 'Oh no, not you. You're too young'. And then the secretary said what address. So she said my old address, and I said, 'No, that's me'. And she said, 'Oh, I'm sorry. I didn't realise you were that old', you know. I forgave her for that.* (Doreen, aged 38, interview, 28 weeks, no genetic tests)

Quasi-comic ingredients in the above scenario include near escape from entanglement (*'getting out'*) in a social fiasco, and heightened embarrassment resulting from a string of misunderstandings. The occurrence of such incidents, however infrequently, provides clear evidence for the existence of a stigmatised identity, socially distant from the normal one with which it was mistaken.

Historical ageing

The concept of historical ageing focuses on the ways in which people position themselves in relation to others who are ageing contemporaneously. It refers to both the broad sweep of historical change which generates psychosocial gaps between the generations, and to the flow of biographical events within an individual's immediate social environment.

Historical and personal ageing are as confounded in relation to parenthood as in cross-sectional research. Parents and children may misunderstand each other both because people change as they grow older, and because societal change makes earlier generations old-fashioned. The extent to which historical changes separate the generations will depend both upon their rate and upon the extent to which parents and children identify with past and current trends. Given the accelerating rapidity of technological and cultural change in contemporary society, parents may age historically at a faster rate at the same time as the rate of biological ageing has slowed down because of overall health improvement. As one respondent put it:

Pregnant woman: *And then* [if too old] *you might be out of touch with them, or what's going on.* (Tracy, aged 38, interview, 29 weeks, serum screening)

The following quotation illustrates the historical fissure which the advent of genetic testing has itself created.

Interviewer: *So how did your mam feel about you and your . . .*
Pregnant woman: *She thinks it's lovely . . . It's happened for a purpose . . . And she doesn't really think me age has got, she doesn't think it would cause any problems, you know.*
Interviewer: *Did you talk to your mum about the amniocentesis?*
Pregnant woman: *No . . .*
Interviewer: *Why do you think that you, that you left your mum out of that?*
Pregnant woman: *Just because, really, I didn't want her to worry. And I don't think she would have really, not that she's old or senile or . . . , I don't think she would have understood completely, you know.* (Hilary, aged 40, interview, 23 weeks, amniocentesis)

Ironically, a genetic technology which defines pregnant women aged over 34 as biologically old also makes them historically young.

As well as considering the timing of parenthood in relation to the march of history, women also took account of their relationships with members of other age cohorts, including peers and parents. The respondent quoted below sought to emulate the relatively low age gap between herself and her own mother because she felt that a smaller age difference would help her to maintain a good relationship with her own child.

Pregnant woman: *Me mam's 49, and I think the* [small] *age difference between me and me mam is nice. I mean I'm really close to me mam.* (Sheila, aged 25, interview, 24 weeks, no genetic tests)

Another woman saw herself as on-time, despite starting a family at a relatively old age, because a family member with whom she had a close relationship had given birth at about the same time.

Pregnant woman: *And last year my brother had a baby, his girlfriend had a baby, and so I think when you have one in the family . . . and having* *one so close, and being involved with her quite a bit, and we thought, 'Right that's it.'* (Pauline, aged 34, interview, 28 weeks, no genetic tests)

This micro-historical temporal congruence overrode any sense of lateness derived from the wider parental social clock.

Age and non-parental roles

Women calibrated their parental age in relation to the chronology of other important roles, particularly marriage and careers. Those who married relatively late sometimes balanced the youth of their marriage against their age as potential parents.

> **Pregnant woman:** *I have been married for 2 years, so, I mean, I haven't known* [husband] *for very long. And I wanted time to, I mean, I actually needed time to accept the fact that, or to get used to the idea that, we might have a child. I wasn't ready earlier.* (Angela, aged 38, interview, 22 weeks, serum screening)

Because she had married relatively late, this respondent felt that she needed time to develop and cement the marital relationship before launching into parenthood.

The tendency for middle-class women to delay the timing of their first pregnancy is well-documented. We found a strong statistical relationship between pregnant women's ages and their socio-economic status in our survey data. Not surprisingly, some women reported that they had delayed parenthood in order to allow time for the development of a 'young' career.

> **Pregnant woman:** *I didn't want to have a baby right after I'd graduated from university and had my job. So I wanted to have some experience as a teacher before I started a family.* (Kate, aged 32, interview, 20 weeks, no genetic tests)

Women working in lower status jobs which lacked career structure would have had no incentive to establish themselves before starting a family. On the other hand, very young parenthood was often criticised on the grounds that the parents would lack the resources needed to support a family:

> **Pregnant woman:** *They can't financially support a family.* (Questionnaire)

The chronologically young are often financially young, although, in areas of mass unemployment, a significant proportion of the population may be condemned to this state for long periods of their lives. Hence, the significance of occupational time depends upon the social organisation of work.

Genetic age

Genetic age derives from the relatively recent finding that the risk of a foetus having Down's syndrome increases with maternal and, to a lesser extent, paternal age. This finding gives rise to a new legitimation for disapproval of older mothering (Nelkin and Tancredi, 1989), the general categorisation of which as a medical problem can be traced back at least to the seventeenth century (Points, 1957).

Some older women accepted the categorisation of them as genetically old.

> **Interviewer:** *Is that* [thinking about amniocentesis] *different this time round, do you think, than with the other pregnancies?*
> **Pregnant woman:** *Yeh, aha, definitely.*
> **Interviewer:** *Why?*
> **Pregnant woman:** *Mainly I think 'cos of me age . . . I mean, I might look it because I'm shattered out, just finished work, but like em, I don't feel 40, if you know what I mean. But I think me age, with being 40, that plays a big part in going for the amnio, you know . . . I think you just, you want reassurance.* (Hilary, aged 40, interview, 23 weeks, amniocentesis)

This respondent had experienced dissonance between her generally youthful apparent and vital ages on the one hand and her elderly genetic status on the other. In contrast, the woman quoted below rejected the categorisation of her as old implicit in the current policy, at our hospital research site, of offering genetic tests to women aged 35 and over.

> **Interviewer:** *Have any of your friends or anybody that you have talked to had testing?*
> **Pregnant woman:** *No. Well, they all had kids young anyway so . . .*
> **Interviewer:** *Are none of them over 35?*
> **Pregnant woman:** *No.*
> **Interviewer:** *And how does that make you feel?*

Pregnant woman: *I don't know. I don't feel 35.* (Heather, aged 36, interview after taped hospital consultation [Bell], 18 weeks, no genetic tests)

The tension between genetic and other ageing chronologies is nicely illustrated by a woman's humorous interjection at the end of her hospital consultation.

Doctor: *One of the things I want you to hang on to and remember is that, despite this terrible age problem . . .*
Pregnant woman: *I am still younger than you.*
Doctor: *You have many, many more chances of being normal than abnormal.* (Linda, aged 39, hospital consultation [Loftus], 12 weeks, amniocentesis)

Because genetic age derived from the risk of giving birth to a baby with Down's syndrome, it could be changed by screening/testing. For example, a serum screening test result would, in effect, make a woman either genetically younger or older, as doctors sometimes pointed out in hospital consultations.

Doctor: *It* [serum screening] *doesn't tell us whether the baby has got Down's syndrome, but it will give us an idea. So it can make your risk maybe go up, for a 40 year old, but bring it down to, maybe, a 23 year old, at which case you would not be discussing any of this at all.* (Sarah, aged 36, hospital consultation [Dickson], 10 weeks, amniocentesis)

If she had accepted serum screening, this respondent would have ended up genetically aged either 23 or 40 in relation to her risk of Down's syndrome.

Genetic ageing took place, for these women, in the context of a selective screening/testing system which targeted those aged 35 and over. This dividing line defined a boundary for becoming genetically old which was organisationally driven, as one pregnant midwife noted.

Pregnant midwife: *Because you are over 35, then you are older, so you are offered screening. But then, maybe, if screening was, if nobody was offered screening until they were 38, then people wouldn't be old until they were 38. And if it was 40, well, you wouldn't be old, you are still young at 38.* (Shirley, midwife, aged 34, interview, 20 weeks, no genetic tests)

Genetic old age was, in this sense, constituted by the screening/testing system. Women who did not see such age boundaries as organisationally driven could view this mysterious boundary as 'magic' even if they accepted it.

> **Pregnant midwife:** *I wasn't ready earlier* [to have children], *but then 36, was the magic mark. In a sense, that's when you start ticking over into the seriously getting old.*
> **Interviewer:** *What does seriously getting old mean to you?*
> **Pregnant woman:** *Abnormalities, is the first thing. Second thing is fatigue, and will you be able to conceive at all?* (Jackie, midwife, aged 36, interview, 14 weeks, no genetic tests)

(See the section on *'Maternal Age as a Binary Risk Marker'* in Chapter 4 for a further discussion.)

Those pregnant women who had crossed this organisationally generated boundary could feel alienated from younger women who had not.

> **Interviewer:** *Have you felt at all that, this is, in a sense that it's a few years since you* [didn't have to worry about genetic decision-making] . . . .
> **Pregnant woman:** *Yes. Oh no, I have felt that you know, especially the girl who said to me at work, you know, 'You want to* [be tested] *because there is enough Down's Syndrome kids in the world anyway.' I felt like punching her, you know. She had three children. She never had to go through this because she is younger than me.* (Marietta, aged 39, interview after hospital consultation [Laughton], 12 weeks, amniocentesis)

Medical age

The notion of genetic age is underpinned by clear inductive evidence of a strong statistical association between maternal age and the risk of giving birth to a baby with Down's syndrome. Women and health professionals could also view maternal older age as a more generally risky condition.

> **Interviewer:** *Did you go to your doctor's appointments with both pregnancies?*
> **Previously pregnant woman:** *Oh yes.*

Interviewer: *Did you go to them all?*
Previously pregnant woman: *Ah yes, I went religiously.*
Interviewer: *Why was that? . . .*
Previously pregnant woman: *Well, I think especially with my age, I think they can do things that can help you, and they can give you advice. They know more about it than I do, so, obviously, I would go to them, and listen to them . . . I feel safe with them.* (Audrey, aged 39, interview, post-partum, serum screening)

This woman's diffuse sense of her age as a medical problem led her to comply *'religiously'* with the requirement to attend antenatal clinics, where, as we saw in Chapter 1, her concerns would have been focused onto age-related genetic risk. Unusually, in the risk society, she trusted the experts, with whom she felt *'safe'*, although this confidence did not extend to her GP, whom she did not *'trust'*.

Pregnant women and health professionals may associate older maternal age with a diffuse, generalised vulnerability to undefined risks. The conclusion that older women do not suffer a greater risk of complications other than age-related genetic abnormalities has been reported a number of times (Mansfield, 1988; Ales, Druzin and Santini, 1990; Berkowitz *et al.*, 1990; Duchon and Muise, 1993). However, recent studies have produced evidence that older women face greater risk of maternal mortality (DOH *et al.*, 1998) than do younger women; and that the risk of foetal loss (Andersen *et al.*, 2000) is associated with maternal age even when the potentially confounding factors of susceptibility to miscarriages and fertility are controlled for. The epidemiological risk picture, tentative and subject to revision, can be differentiated from the cultural representation of older pregnant women as a generically high-risk group.

Whilst some women accepted their high-risk status, others resented the way in which the highlighting of genetic risk and other possibly age-related risks defined them as old.

Pregnant woman: *No they didn't mention it* [maternal age] *last time, but this time they did. To be quite honest, I came out feeling more like 58 rather than 38. And after a lot of soul searching I just decided not to bother with anything.* (Diane, aged 38, interview, 16 weeks, no genetic tests)

A few respondents felt positively stigmatised for placing themselves in the medical category of older pregnant woman.

Pregnant woman: *I went back, and I waited to see another midwife. And I said, 'I've got a water specimen'. And she tested it, and it was. But I had been feeling tired and listless and drowsy, and I'd had pains in my side. And she said to me, 'Well, you're old, your muscles have not got back into shape', and, you know, 'It's your muscles stretching.' And I said, 'Well, excuse me, but I thought muscles were supposed to stretch.' And by that time I was thinking, 'Ah, I just don't need this. I don't need to be told I'm old.'* (Doreen, aged 38, interview, 28 weeks, no genetic tests)

The woman quoted below felt that health professionals had employed tactful labelling in order to minimise the social distance between herself and younger women.

Interviewer: *Have you been conscious of your age at all?*
Pregnant woman: *Do you mean with the midwives at the hospital or just in general?*
Interviewer: *In general.*
Pregnant woman: *Yeah in general, but not at the hospital or the mid-wives. They haven't really singled me out much from the other women, but I'm classed as what you call a 'mature' mother.* (Patricia, aged 37, inter-view, 24 weeks, serum screening)

Sensitive professionals take care with the labelling of potentially stigmatised identities. The above respondent suggested that a euphemism was being used to spare her feelings. Such efforts can reinforce stigmatisation if the recipient realises that an awkward topic is being skirted round. They also leave the grounds for the initial classification of older pregnancy as a serious medical problem taken for granted.

Evidence of the overall impact of perceived medical risk on value judgements about parental age also comes from the one survey finding of a statistically significant relationship between these judgements and reasons given for them. The mean age at which a woman was judged too old to have a baby was lower among women who mentioned medical risk (42.0 years) than among those who did not (44.3 years). The difference is highly statistically significant ($F_{1,388} = 22.3$, $P < 0.001$) with respondent age and socio-economic status controlled for.

Reasons for parental age judgements

Analysis of the survey data provides a quantitative overview of respondents' reasoning about age limits for parenthood which summarises

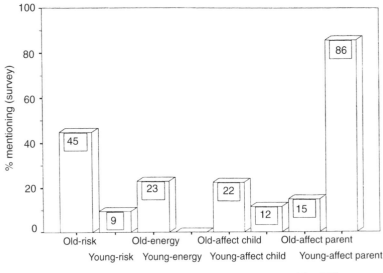

N (Why woman too young) = 698; N (Why woman too old) = 585

Figure 2.2　Why is a Woman too Old or Young to Have a Baby?

much of the material discussed above. Those who agreed that a man or woman could be too old or too young to have a baby were invited to give reasons for their judgements through replying to an open-ended question. The reasons given were grouped, and the reliability of these categories checked through blind coding of a sample of responses by an independent judge. An agreement level of better than 90 per cent was obtained. The results are summarised in Figure 2.2 for reasons why a woman might be too young or old to have a baby.

A similar profile was found for men, except that, as would be expected, very few explanations of why a man could be too old to become a parent referred to medical risks. Reasons were given by 72 per cent (585) of the 807 respondents who believed that a woman could be too old, and by 61 per cent (698) of the 1149 respondents who thought that a woman could be too young, to have a baby.

Explanations have been grouped into the four categories shown in Figure 2.2. Those involving medical risk to the mother and/or baby, lack of maternal energy and adverse effects on the child were offered more frequently with respect to why women were thought too old to have a baby. In contrast, women were considered too young primarily because of adverse effects on the mother, for example that she would miss out on enjoyable social activities. Hence, mothers were thought too old primarily because of the presumed damaging effects on the child, and too young because of the anticipated negative consequences for the mother. We have seen that both older and younger pregnant women challenge the implicit stereotypes about their needs and capabilities on which age norms about parenting are based.

3
The Offer of Genetic Screening/Testing

Introduction

The next five chapters will explore the operation of genetic screening and testing at our hospital research site. This chapter will consider the question of who was offered genetic screening and testing, a necessary precursor of women exercising choice, since women could only select from the options which they identified as available to them. The next two chapters will focus on women's decisions about genetic screening/testing. Chapters 6 and 7 will examine in some detail the complex issues discussed during the brief six to seven-minute hospital consultations in which a doctor advised selected women about genetic screening/testing options.

The preventative system which women were asked to navigate is mapped in Figure 3.1.

The hospital doctors to whom we presented this diagram were struck by its complexity, and requested simplification. However, it represents the decision maze which women have to navigate. Even if doctors block off some of the possible routes through the system by only offering particular choices of genetic tests, women may realise, as we shall see, that a different doctor might have opened up other pathways. The diagram puts into perspective the well-established finding that women's understanding of the genetic screening/testing system for Down's syndrome is often limited (Smith *et al.*, 1994; Marteau, 1995). Smith *et al.* found that less than 40 per cent of their sample of women who had received serum screening for Down's syndrome realised that this was the main purpose of the test, understood that most women who test positive have normal babies, or appreciated that negative results did not guarantee perfect health in other respects. Improved information-giving may

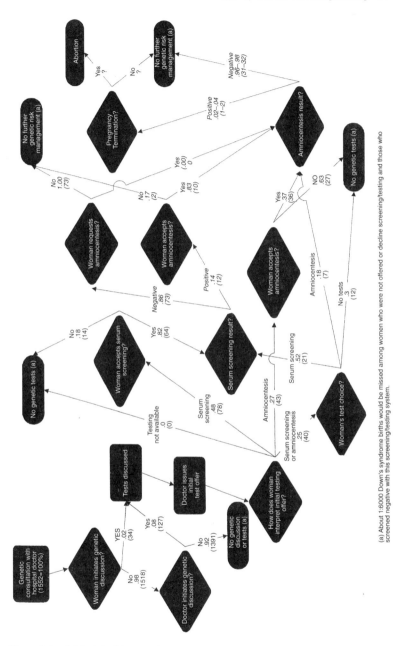

Figure 3.1 A Model of Prenatal Genetic Decision-Making Based on Survey Data (N = 1552). (*Estimated statistics in italics*)

mitigate this alarming level of misunderstanding, which makes a mockery of informed choice. However, the inherent difficulty of the task of explaining a preventative system as complex as that represented in Figure 3.1 has not been sufficiently acknowledged.

An attempt has been made to estimate the numerical flow of the sample through the genetic decision-taking maze. The numbers cannot all be taken literally, as some, shown in italics, had to be extrapolated from other data. But the flow-diagram does provide a fairly accurate picture of the proportions taking different routes through the genetic screening/testing system at our hospital research site. This picture cannot be generalised to other hospitals since the decisions which women took depended upon what they were offered. This, in turn, was contingent on the policies and practice of both the hospital and individual doctors. Hence, Figure 3.1 offers an analysis of how one maternity hospital and the pregnant women who gave birth there together managed certain targeted genetic risks.

Although the reader may feel slightly bewildered by the complexity of Figure 3.1, it offers only a general map of the decision-making landscape which women were required to navigate. Each of the decision points shown required consideration of a complex, interrelated set of issues. For example, women who were offered amniocentesis had to decide: whether they would be willing to terminate their pregnancy if an abnormality was discovered; if so, whether the perceived risk of miscarriage outweighed the chance of giving birth to a genetically abnormal baby; and, if they were not willing to terminate, whether they would still wish to obtain information before the birth about the genetic status of the foetus.

Joining the maze

As will be shown below, the survey data suggested that the most important determinants of a woman's selection of genetic screening/testing options were whether it was discussed with the hospital doctor at the consultation which all women received; and, if so, which forms of test were offered. With respect to the former decision, only 2% (34) of women who completed the survey indicated that they had requested advice about genetic screening/testing. In the other 98 per cent of cases, hospital doctors decided whether screening/testing should be discussed. A further 8 per cent (127) of the survey sample indicated that the hospital doctor had initiated a discussion of genetic screening/testing. Analysis of a sample of 231 records also showed that about

10 per cent of pregnant women attending the hospital were offered genetic tests.

We have already noted, in the Introduction, that hospital consultants would have liked to offer Down's syndrome screening/testing combined with advice from a trained genetic counsellor to all women, but had been refused the necessary funding. If a substantially higher proportion of women had themselves requested such advice, doctors would have been faced with a choice between refusal, thus violating the principle of consumer choice, and unmanageable extra demands on their own time. An additional 18 per cent (277) of the survey sample indicated that they would have liked to have been given genetic screening/testing choice. Hence, the smooth operation of the overall system of prenatal genetic risk management required that only a small proportion of women should themselves ask about genetic tests.

Socio-economic status and requesting genetic tests

Discussion of genetic screening/testing at one's own request was significantly associated with women's socio-economic status. With maternal age statistically controlled for, women of higher socio-economic status were 4.4 times likelier (95 per cent confidence intervals = 1.3–14.9) than those of lower status to report having asked about genetic screening/testing ($P = 0.02$). This finding suggests that hospital responsiveness to women's own wishes may have unintentionally created social inequality in access to rationed services. With maternal age controlled for, women of higher socio-economic status were 1.6 times likelier (95 per cent confidence intervals = 1.0–2.5) than those of lower status to indicate that they had been offered genetic tests ($P = 0.04$). When respondents who reported asking about screening/testing were excluded from the analysis, this relationship was reduced and became statistically insignificant.

The offer of genetic screening

Having engaged in discussion of genetic screening/testing with the hospital doctor, women found themselves presented with various test options. We have divided this process into two analytic steps: firstly, the doctor issues a genetic screening/testing offer; and, secondly, the woman interprets this offer. This separation is required because a pregnant woman's understanding of the options available may not correspond to the message which the doctor intended to convey.

When is an offer really an offer?

Yes/no answers to a survey question cover up the processes of interpretation through which women assess the underlying status of an offer of genetic tests. Qualitative analysis illuminates these processes, particularly when, as in the last two examples discussed in this section, the dialogue in the hospital consultation can be compared with a woman's interpretation of what she had been told.

The doctor quoted below emphasised both the low risk of Down's syndrome for younger women and the disadvantages of serum screening before more or less offering genetic tests.

> **Doctor:** *Your risk for sporadic Down's is 1 in 1210. If you were 37, it is 1 in 240. So, there is quite a dramatic change in that 10 years, and it is really that sort of age group, as I say, about 30s onwards, that's the area, that's the age group we target . . . We tend, we have taken a deliberate decision, it's not related to funding or anything like that . . . to target rather than do it for everybody because we know that it can generate a tremendous amount of heartache if you get a false positive and so on. And there would be further tests . . . , sometimes amniocentesis, where there is an actual real risk of that in relation to termination of the pregnancy* (Lucy, aged 27, hospital consultation [Loftus], 12 weeks, no genetic tests)

The form of the offer of serum screening made its acceptance difficult. The woman's risk of Down's syndrome was framed in relation to the higher risks faced by older women, and categorised as *'pretty low'*; the financial cost of the procedure within a resource-limited NHS was hinted at; and the iatrogenic risks arising from false positives were spelt out.

The next quotation shows how a screening/testing option could be virtually ruled out as inappropriate even though its technical availability was acknowledged.

> **Pregnant woman:** *I think, well there's more risk of having a Down's baby over 35, isn't there? . . . But [hospital doctor] said, 'I'm not even going to offer you the blood test because it might lead you into a false sense of security, and we know you're high risk' . . . So that threw us a bit, 'cos I thought, 'Oh, it's only a matter of the blood test. I'll probably not have to have the other one.' But, I don't know, it was just a lot more worrying than I thought it would be.* (Beatrice, aged 40, interview, 26 weeks, amniocentesis)

This woman, like the last respondent quoted, did not appear to resent this restriction of choice, but interpreted it as an indicator of the seriousness of the risk she faced. Another woman, of a similar age, had not even realised that she could have opted for serum screening until she read about it after undergoing amniocentesis.

> **Interviewer:** *Did you think about the blood test at all? Did you know about the blood test?*
> **Pregnant woman:** *No. Em, which one?*
> **Interviewer:** *The triple test.*
> **Pregnant woman:** *The triple test, no. Em, I didn't know about that until after. I read in the books, and I thought, well, it does say that it's not available in some areas. And I thought, 'Oh, I've had the tests now, it doesn't matter' . . . not that we were given the choice or anything. . . .*
> **Interviewer:** *Did you feel any pressure to have the test?*
> **Pregnant woman:** *Oh no, no. It was our decision.* (Gemma, aged 41, interview, 38 weeks, amniocentesis)

The above respondent had not realised that she could have opted for serum screening as an alternative to amniocentesis. She felt untroubled by this lack of choice when it was pointed out, and assumed that serum screening had not been offered because of its inappropriateness for women of her age. Nevertheless, she had been denied an option which, otherwise, she might have considered. We will argue below that a strategy of steering the oldest, highest risk women towards amniocentesis, the more accurate, but also more invasive alternative, increased the probability that these women would not undergo any form of test.

In two cases, follow-up interviews allowed us to assess the impact of doctors' specific advice on women's perceptions of the choices available. These two contrasting examples illustrate the different ways in which women actively interpreted genetic test offers.

Her doctor offered the woman quoted below an explicit choice of both available tests.

> **Doctor:** *As I say, the choices are yours. You may decide you want to do nothing, you may decide you want to have the blood test, or you may decide you want to just leave it, or have the fluid away from around the baby* [amniocentesis]. (Margaret, aged 35, hospital consultation [Anderson], 14 weeks, serum screening.)

However, the doctor warned this woman that with amniocentesis, *'obviously, you have to accept then that you have greater risk of miscarrying a normal baby than you have of us detecting a child with a problem'.* Moreover, the portrayal of amniocentesis as having *'the fluid away'* suggests drastic surgery, akin to amputation.

At the end of the consultation, she asked for further information, and was offered a leaflet on serum screening, which had just been discussed, but not on amniocentesis. In the follow-up interview, this woman stated she had only been offered serum screening. In contrast, the younger woman quoted below agonised about whether to accept serum screening even though the doctor presented this option in a way which made acceptance appear irrational.

> **Doctor:** *I was led to believe that you might be interested in serum screening. Is that right? I mean, the serum screening is really, that's not really, well it's for trisomy, though, so I don't think this is appropriate.* (Elizabeth, aged 25, hospital consultation [Fallowfield], 12 weeks, no genetic tests)

The code switch to trisomy, the genetic cause of Down's syndrome, may have been used to distance the risk of the condition which was usually referred to as Down's syndrome. Was this woman 'offered' genetic tests? The entire content of the session argued against acceptance of the option she had formally been given, and she would have needed considerable determination to opt for serum screening. Nevertheless, her comments in a follow-up interview showed that she had treated serum screening as a serious option.

> **Pregnant woman:** . . . *and then* [hospital doctor] *put it to me that if I said I wanted these tests, that I had to make sure that if I got the result that I didn't want I would have to make a decision about that. So did I want to know, or did I not want to know? So it was really a slap in the face. And there was no, sort of, you know, 'But don't worry, these cases are* [rare]'. *There was nothing to cushion the blow. And that was at nine weeks. And I was really, it was a shock pregnancy anyway. I was away from home. My family live in Wales. It was awful.* (Elizabeth, aged 25, interview after taped hospital consultation [Fallowfield], 13 weeks, no genetic tests)

The dynamics of this instructive episode can be unpacked as follows. The doctor intended to convey a reassuring risk message, that at age 25, this woman's probability of Down's syndrome did not warrant genetic screening/testing. The doctor offered genetic screening as an option that she was entitled to, but which was unnecessary. However, risk consciousness, heightened by the shock of an unplanned pregnancy and the remoteness of family support, prevented this woman from absorbing the doctor's reassuring message. She then interpreted the doctor's non-mention of her low risk of bearing a baby with Down's syndrome as indicative of an unsupportive approach. But the doctor, probably, had not appreciated that attempting to rule out genetic screening had alarmed her.

Hospital genetic tests offers

Figure 3.1 provides an overview of the genetic tests offered to our survey sample. Only a quarter of the 10 per cent (161) of the survey sample who reported having been offered any genetic tests stated that they had been given a choice of test. Within this sub-sample, 48 per cent (78) said that they had been offered serum screening, 27 per cent (43) amniocentesis, and 25 per cent (40) a choice of either test. The age distribution of women who received genetic screening/testing offers is depicted in Figure 3.2.

Not surprisingly, Figure 3.2 demonstrates that screening/testing was clearly targeted at older, higher risk women; and that older women were particularly likely to be offered the more accurate, but also more problematic option of amniocentesis. However, 28 per cent (30) of women

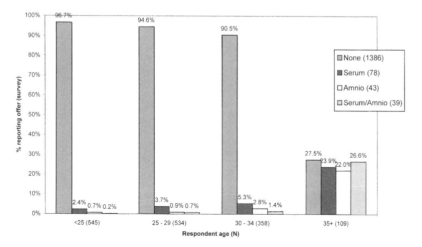

Figure 3.2   Genetic Testing Offers by Age Group (N = 1546)

aged 35 and over reported not being offered either serum screening or amniocentesis. And 6 per cent (81) of younger women were also offered tests. Women's perceptions of the choices available to them (serum screening, amniocentesis or either test) will be discussed further below.

The impact of offering tests to younger women on the overall age distribution of screening/testing at our hospital research site can be seen in Figure 3.3.

Although women aged under 35 were less likely to be offered tests, a substantial proportion of test offers, including two-thirds of offers of serum screening only, went to the younger age group, simply because a large majority of pregnant women (93 per cent of our survey sample) were aged under 35.

Genetic screening/testing offers were directed to substantial numbers of women well below the official, but not precisely defined, high-risk boundary of around 35. Two arguments against this conclusion can be put forward: firstly, that younger women were selected because of a family history of Down's syndrome or other chromosomal conditions; and, secondly, that younger women may have confused genetic with other tests, over-reporting the extent to which they had been offered.

In rebuttal of the family history explanation of the above findings, it can be pointed out that the rate of screening/testing offers to women aged under 35 was much higher than could be explained in terms of the prevalence of family histories of genetic abnormalities. Moreover, exclusion from the analysis of women who mentioned such histories

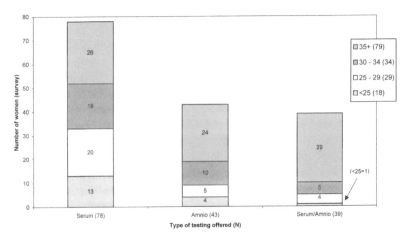

Figure 3.3   Age Group by Offers of Genetic Testing (N = 160)

from the survey analysis reduced the proportion of women under 35 who reported having been offered genetic tests, from 6 per cent (81) to 4 per cent (58), but still left a substantial number of genetic test offers to be explained. Twelve respondents aged under 35 without a history of Down's syndrome reported having been offered amniocentesis but not serum screening.

In relation to the second rebuttal, that our evidence relies on women's perceptions, we have already noted that statistics obtained from hospital records matched those derived from our survey quite closely. The following quotation, from a pregnant midwife, illustrates the apparently *ad hoc* nature of doctors' decisions about offering genetic tests.

Pregnant Midwife: *If they* [pregnant women] *have thought about screening they usually mention something to you. And at 33* [pregnant woman's age], *I thought, it is not my position to actually mention screening. Usually, if they are 35 you will say, 'Well, have you considered screening?' . . . But this registrar had actually offered screening. I think she* [pregnant woman] *got quite a shock, because I don't think she really expected, and then I think she went ahead with the screening without thinking what the consequence was like . . . I kept thinking, should I have said something to prepare her? But then again, is it my job to do this you see? It is difficult. You don't know what to do.* (Shirley, midwife, aged 34, interview, 20 weeks, no genetic tests)

Because midwives could not fully anticipate which women would be offered screening/testing, they could not know whom to prepare in advance of the medical consultation. The quotation also illustrates the uninformed way in which pregnant women had to decide about, and usually accepted, serum screening, without regard to its consequences.

The maternal age distribution for genetic screening/testing at our hospital research site was affected by the competing influences of current 'evidence-based' and 'consumer choice' ideologies. Doctors responded to the former by directing their limited screening/testing resources towards older women, the higher risk group. At the same time, the conflicting injunction to take account of the perspectives of service users led them to offer genetic tests to younger, lower risk women whom they felt might welcome them.

The absence of genetic test offers to 28 per cent (30) of women aged 35 and over can also be partly explained in terms of doctors' responsiveness to their preferences. Among 24 of the 30 women aged over 34 who answered this question, 14 (58 per cent) indicated that they had not wanted to be offered genetic tests. The other 10 women (42 per cent), who reported that they would have liked to have been offered genetic screening/testing, had slipped through the preventative net despite being classified into the higher risk group. A small number of these women may not have been offered genetic tests because they had passed the appropriate gestational age range. However, out of five of these ten women who suggested reasons why they might not have been offered genetic tests, only one thought that it was because the hospital consultation occurred too late in her pregnancy. Three believed that they were not at the right age, or that the hospital considered genetic tests unnecessary, and one woman did not know the reason.

When we discussed this finding with groups of hospital doctors, they agreed that omission of maternal age from a woman's case notes could lead to her higher risk status being overlooked. One doctor suggested that this procedural error might occur in a number of circumstances: if the woman looked younger than her age; if distracted by another, pressing clinical concern; or even if the phone rang. Another pointed out that women aged over 34 who gave birth to babies with Down's syndrome had successfully sued a hospital which had not offered them genetic tests. The apparently simple policy of offering genetic screening/testing to all women aged over 34 turned out to be not so easy to translate into organisational practice.

Who was offered genetic screening/testing?

As already stated (see Figure 3.1), 2 per cent (34) of the survey sample discussed genetic screening/testing in the hospital consultation at their own request, whilst the hospital doctor raised this topic with a further 8 per cent (127) of respondents. Multivariate analysis, via logistic regression, was used to explore the question of why some women were offered advice about genetic screening/testing whilst others were not.

The model outlined below predicts whether a woman was offered either or both available forms of genetic test, serum screening and amniocentesis. Factors associated with the likelihood of being given a particular type of screening/testing option will be considered subsequently. The following variables were included in the initial model: maternal age, socio-economic and marital status (including cohabiting); the number of times the respondent had previously been pregnant; whether she reported any problems in her previous pregnancies; and whether she was concerned about the health of the baby or her own health. Statistically significant relationships are summarised in Table 3.1, and then discussed below.

Statistical interactions were insignificant, and have been eliminated from the model presented in Table 3.1, and discussed below. The analysis generated a two-stage model, in which the probability of women reporting that they had been offered genetic screening/testing was significantly associated with them being older, more concerned about the health of the baby, and of higher socio-economic status. Being concerned about the health of the baby was, in turn, itself related to respondents' concern about her own health, experience of problems in previous pregnancies and higher socio-economic status. Finally, a woman's concern about her own health was not statistically associated

Table 3.1 Predictors of Offers of Genetic Screening or Testing and Co-variables

Being offered genetic screening or testing (N = 1255)

Maternal predictor	N	Odds (95% confidence intervals)	Probability
Age			0.000
< = 30	830	1	
31–34	325	1.9 (1.1–3.2)	0.01
35+	100	57.3 (31.2–102.2)	0.000
Concerned for health of baby			
No	1028	1	
Yes	227	3.0 (1.9–4.9)	0.000
Socio-economic status			
Lower	597	1	
Higher	658	2.0 (1.2–3.3)	0.005

Concerned about the health of the baby (N = 1236)

Maternal predictor	N	Odds (95% confidence intervals)	Probability
Concern about own health			
No	1104	1	
Yes	132	3.0 (2.0–4.6)	0.000
Previous pregnancy problems			
No	926	1	
Yes	310	2.6 (1.9–3.5)	0.000
Socio-economic status			
Lower	584	1	
Higher	652	2.3 (1.7–3.2)	0.000

with other demographic variables, including maternal age, and marital and socio-economic status. It must be pointed out, however, that an Australian study (Searle, 1996) found no relationship between mothers' anxiety about their baby having abnormalities and socio-economic status. As well as employing a smaller sample, this study focused on only one source of risk consciousness. Ours detected a relationship between maternal socio-economic status and overall concern about the baby's health.

Not surprisingly, in view of the hospital's selective screening policy, women aged 35 and over were about 50 times more likely to report being offered genetic tests than were those below this arbitrary but entrenched risk dividing line. The marginal risk status of women aged 30–34 is reflected in their intermediate odds, as they were about twice as likely as younger women to be offered genetic tests. Women who were concerned about the health of their baby were three times more likely to be offered genetic tests than those who were not. Those of higher socio-economic status (who owned their own homes and had access to a car) were twice as likely to be offered genetic tests as women from poorer backgrounds. However, exclusion of the 2 per cent (34) of respondents who had asked about genetic tests eliminated this relationship, but not that between being offered genetic tests and concern for the health of the baby, from the model. This finding suggests that, on aggregate, more prosperous women were better able to mobilise health service resources, by requesting and receiving services, if they wished to do so. Overall, women of higher socio-economic status who were concerned about the health of their baby were about four times more likely (odds ratio = 3.9, 95 per cent confidence intervals = 2.2–6.8) than poorer, unworried women to be offered genetic tests.

The above findings can be explained on the basis that a heightened but diffuse risk consciousness, associated directly or indirectly with concern about one's own health or that of the baby, previous pregnancy problems and socio-economic status, triggers the preventative response of being offered genetic tests. This process coexists with the evidence-based consideration of maternal age. As we shall show below, women's heightened risk consciousness invoked this preventative response even where, as in most cases, their concerns were unrelated to genetic issues. Additionally (see Table 3.3), signs of maternal concern increased the probability not only that women would be offered tests, but also that they would be offered amniocentesis, the 'heavier' of the two test options. In effect, their worry, whatever its source, caused women to be treated as genetically older than their chronological age.

Further analysis showed that a woman's 'risk' of being offered genetic tests increased if she was concerned about the health of her baby regardless of the focus of her anxiety. The above logistic regression analysis was repeated with a sub-sample of respondents, 6 per cent (87) of the total, who were particularly concerned about genetic issues, excluded from the analysis. Members of this sub-sample explained their concern with the health of their baby in terms of its genetic normality, indicated that a previous child had been born with an abnormality, or mentioned a family history of genetic problems. The statistical relationship between the probability of being offered genetic tests and concern for the health of the baby was reduced only slightly by their exclusion. Women worried about the health of their baby for non-genetic reasons were 2.2 times more likely than those who were not to be offered genetic tests (P = 0.005), with maternal age controlled for. This odds ratio is only slightly less than that of 3.0, obtained for the entire sample, as shown in Table 3.1.

This finding suggests that pregnant women and hospital staff identified risk consciousness globally rather than in terms of specific problems. A similar trend was found for each of the seven registrars and consultants whose clients were included in the survey, indicating that all were more likely to offer genetic tests to women who were worried about the health of their baby. The offer of a test was likely to be accepted, regardless of a woman's age, at least in the case of serum screening, as will be shown below. It can be concluded that women who had any health concerns about their baby, for example, about its position in the womb, were more likely both to be offered, and to accept, genetic tests.

We will attempt to justify below the causal assumption that their heightened risk consciousness resulted in women being more likely to be offered genetic tests. Taking the direction of causality, temporarily, for granted allows us to identify an example of a perhaps more general process of risk abstraction. Human service organisations may respond to clients' specific worries about the future by classifying these concerns as exemplars of risk, and then responding by delivering those protective measures which they are mobilised to provide. Risk concern is met by protection even though their foci are causally unconnected. Qualitative support for this proposition will be offered below.

The causal direction of the relationship between a woman's concern for the health of the baby and the probability of her being offered genetic screening cannot be inferred from cross-sectional data. This association may have arisen because both of the above variables were associated with a third, unknown factor. Any direct causal influence might work in two directions. Medical staff may attempt to help anxious women by offering tests, as we have argued, or, alternatively, the offer of tests may increase their anxiety. Both processes may occur, with initial anxiety increasing women's chances of being offered tests, and such offers further heightening their anxiety. The qualitative data analysed in Chapter 5 will illustrate the latter process.

Evidence that women's anxiety may have stimulated doctors, consciously or unconsciously, to offer genetic tests comes from analysis of the views of those who were not offered them. Table 3.2 presents a comparable analysis to that provided in Table 3.1, but with reference to predictors of whether women who were not offered genetic tests would have liked to have received this option.

As shown in Table 3.2, women who were concerned about the health of their baby, and those aged over 34 were significantly more likely to wish they had been offered genetic tests than the remainder, in each case, of the sample. Since genetic screening/testing had not been mentioned to these women, their concern about the health of their baby cannot have resulted from having been designated as eligible. Moreover, as found for offers of genetic tests, exclusion from the analysis of women who expressed specifically genetic concerns did not affect this relationship. This finding provides supporting evidence for the proposition that worried women were more likely to welcome genetic tests regardless of the source of their worry. Doctors may have sensed and responded to this need. However, engagement in the process of genetic screening and testing is unlikely to have a calming effect, and may heighten a concerned woman's anxiety still further.

Table 3.2   Predictors of Regretting not Having Been Offered Genetic Screening or Testing (N = 1059)

Predictor	N	Odds (95% confidence intervals)	Probability
Age			
<35	779	1	
35+	280	2.3 (1.0–5.4)	0.04
Concerned about health of baby			
No	888	1	
Yes	171	2.2 (1.6–3.1)	0.000

Qualitative evidence

Hospital doctors with whom we discussed this finding readily agreed that they might respond to cues indicating that a woman was worried by offering genetic screening/testing. According to their own accounts, one doctor felt inhibited from probing about the reasons for women's anxiety, particularly in a consultation which could only last for a few minutes; whilst another attempted to reassure a woman worried about an unrelated matter, for example the effect of medication on the baby, by offering genetic tests.

The quotations which follow illustrate the way in which a woman's concern about her own health and that of the baby could become linked, generating a diffuse sense of heightened risk consciousness which the hospital might respond to by offering genetic tests. The first woman cited linked her age, work stress and worry about the pregnancy outcome.

> **Pregnant woman:** *'Cos I mean, not last week, but the week before, I'd been to work, and I was late, and I finished at nine o'clock. And, em, we had a really heavy shift, it was really heavy, and I come home, went in the bath, come downstairs, went to bed . . . And I was a bit frightened then when I went to bed. And I thought, 'Ee, I hope I haven't done, em, any damage or anything', you know, but I was alright the next day, you know. I think it must have just been over-tiredness, you know. I think it is age.*
> (Hilary, aged 40, interview, 23 weeks, amniocentesis)

This woman linked the fragility, as she saw it, of her own health to a generalised concern about *'anything'* happening to the baby. The next respondent contrasted her present state of anxiety with the lesser worry which she experienced when pregnant at a younger age.

> **Pregnant woman:** *I know that if anything happens, I won't go in for another one at the age I am now, and especially with the trouble I've had with these veins, that I would be really upset, especially now. So, I think I've worried about that a little bit more, whereas me second pregnancy, with [girl's name], I worried 'till I got to about 16 weeks, and then I thought, 'Oh well, nothing can happen now.' I wasn't worried after that, where, this time, you realise, and you hear more, that it can happen.*
> (Denise, aged 36, interview, 32 weeks, no genetic tests).

The quotation brings out two qualitative differences between the anxiety which this woman experienced at a younger and older age.

Firstly, the latter fear had lasted for a longer period, and could be expected to continue right through the pregnancy. Secondly, this respondent's concern about the progress of the pregnancy became bound up with her appraisal of her general health. Few women separated their genetic and general health in the way which is articulated in the next quotation.

> **Pregnant woman:** *And she* [respondent's mother] *kept saying, 'It will be alright. I don't know why you think it won't be alright. And everybody else's baby in the family's been alright. And everybody's healthy.' I don't think she understood, really . . . Well, I felt like saying, 'Well it's got nothing to do with whether I'm healthy or not' . . . 'Cos I thought, 'Oh, she doesn't realise.' It's like a chromosome thing, isn't it?* (Beatrice, aged 40, interview, 26 weeks, amniocentesis)

The above respondent pointed out that the grandmother had conflated the mother's general health with the genetic health of the baby. Lippman (1999) found, in a qualitative study of older Canadian pregnant women, that some similarly conflated genetic and wider health risks. They reasoned that their general fitness reduced their vulnerability to all forms of health risk, including genetic ones. This form of reasoning is based on induction. In general, people who feel healthy are less likely to suffer specific diseases. Although the proposed link between the mother's health and the genetic normality of the baby lacks epidemiological validity, it fits with current holistic notions of health.

Other women drew comfort from their adherence to the health promotion line. This consideration may have contributed to the decision of the next woman quoted to opt for serum screening, rather than amniocentesis, at the relatively old age of 38.

> **Pregnant woman:** *I mean, I think if you take it to women when they get to 50, and things like that, it's a lot different, you know. But, I mean, I think, if you're fairly fit, healthy, you know, I'm not on any medication, I don't even take headache tablets . . . I don't smoke, I don't drink, so, I might have the occasional glass, you know. But, er, to that extent, I don't really worry about anything like that.* (Tracy, aged 38, interview, 29 weeks, serum screening)

The reasoning behind this instructive quotation can be unpacked as follows. If age is assumed to be a source of risk for older pregnant women, then measures taken to slow the ageing process may ameliorate its effects. The survey results suggest that women did tend to link general health and specific genetic risks in this way.

Genetic screening/testing options

This section will discuss the specific genetic screening/testing choices which women reported having been given. At our hospital research site, women might be offered serum screening, amniocentesis or a choice of either test. As can be seen in Figure 3.1, only 25 per cent (40) of the 161 women with whom genetic screening/testing was discussed reported receiving a choice of either test. Three-quarters of women who were offered genetic tests judged that they had not been able to decide for themselves which of the two available tests to take.

Statistical analysis of associations between respondent characteristics and screening/testing options in the survey data threw up two relationships. Among survey respondents offered tests, older women and those who were concerned about the health of their baby were significantly more likely to be offered a choice of serum screening or amniocentesis, and significantly less likely to be offered serum screening alone. The latter finding is summarised in Table 3.3.

The relationships presented in Table 3.3 partly match those found for being offered genetic tests, as shown in Table 3.1. Younger women, and those who did not express concern about the health of their baby, were more likely to be given the sole option of serum screening if tests were offered. The relationship between socio-economic status and only being offered serum screening was not statistically significant.

Table 3.3 Predictors of Being Offered Serum Screening only among Survey Respondents Offered Tests (N = 158)

Predictor	N	Odds (95% confidence intervals)	Probability
Age			0.0002
35+	77	1	
31–34	34	2.7 (1.1–6.2)	0.02
<30	47	5.5 (2.4–12.5)	0.0001
Concerned for health of baby			
Yes	56	1	
No	102	2.4 (1.2–4.1)	0.02

The age finding can be readily explained in terms of the belief, held by most doctors, that the additional risk associated with amniocentesis was not justified for younger women. Women who expressed concern about the health of their baby were, like older women, less likely to report being offered the sole option of serum screening. Again, exclusion of women who were specifically concerned about, or had a history of, genetic problems, did not affect this pattern of relationships. Putting these findings together with those reported above, it can be concluded that older women, and those who were concerned about the health of their baby, were both more likely to be offered genetic tests, and, if such an offer was made, to be given the more intense option of amniocentesis. Additionally, we will show in Chapter 4 that worried women were less likely to accept serum screening and possibly more likely to accept amniocentesis if offered. In effect, a woman's own heightened risk consciousness, regardless of its source, caused her to be treated as genetically older than her biological age.

Doctors were not solely operating a population-based screening system based on risk factors, as proposed by Castel (1991), but merged this strategy with case-based sensitivity to women's personal concerns. Only time will tell whether the hybrid nature of this approach arises from the transitional status of health-care systems which are gradually shifting towards orientation to populations; or whether the treatment of cases as equivalent members of risk categories can be taken only so far in individualistic Western cultures.

4
Women's Decisions about Genetic Tests I: Values and Probabilities

Introduction

Women could only choose from the genetic screening/testing options, if any, which they had been offered, or, more unusually in our study population, had successfully requested. In the next two chapters, we will first describe the choices which women made; and then analyse their decision-making with reference to both quantitative associations and their own accounts of the reasoning which underlay their choices. This first chapter will discuss the survey findings about women's choices, and then use evidence of associations between these choices and other variables to provide clues about the processes on which they were based. Previous survey-style research into parental decisions about genetic tests, reviewed by Shiloh (1996), has shown that they are influenced by utilitarian considerations, including: aversion to abortion (Wertz *et al.*, 1992); assessment of the severity of Down's syndrome and judgements about the uncertainty-reducing value of genetic tests (Sagi *et al.*, 1992); the degree of risk and desire to have children (Frets *et al.*, 1990). Our survey analysis will add two variables to the list of influencing factors, namely a woman's level of risk consciousness, as indexed by her concern for her own health, and the genetic screening/testing choices which she sees as available to her. Identification of the latter influencing factor brings into consideration the organisational context which determines the menu of available choices.

This survey analysis will be followed by an exploration, based primarily on qualitative data, of the value judgements and beliefs about probability which women drew upon when they made genetic screening/testing decisions. In the next chapter, we will analyse women's temporal considerations; and, finally, discuss the impact on them of genetic screening and testing outcomes. The material has been divided into two chapters solely for convenience. Chapters 4 and 5 offer a detailed quantitative and qualitative analysis of pregnant women's decision-making about genetic screening/testing in one maternity hospital.

The take-up of genetic screening/testing

The decisions made by women who were offered genetic tests, as shown in Figure 3.1, can be summarised as follows. Of 161 women offered amniocentesis and/or serum screening, 67 per cent (108) underwent at least one of these tests. Amniocentesis was much less likely than serum screening to be accepted. Overall, 72 per cent (85) of respondents were serum screened if this test was offered (or, more accurately, they identified it as being offered) either as their sole option or within a menu which included amniocentesis. In contrast, only 28 per cent (23) of women initially offered amniocentesis, with or without the alternative of serum screening, underwent this test. This difference in acceptance rate can be readily explained in terms of the perceived adverse consequences of amniocentesis which entailed an invasive procedure, insertion of a needle into the abdomen, and a possibly increased risk of miscarriage of a healthy foetus. (We have excluded from this statistic ten women, 12 per cent of the 85 serum-screened respondents, who underwent amniocentesis following a positive serum screening result.)

As can be seen in Figure 3.1, women were more likely to accept either test if they believed it was the only option available. Serum screening was taken up by 82 per cent (64), and amniocentesis by 37 per cent (16) of women who saw it as their only option, but by only 52 per cent (21) and 18 per cent (7) respectively of women who thought they could choose either screening/testing option. This finding will be discussed further below (see Table 4.1).

Factors associated with decisions about genetic tests

The take-up of serum screening and amniocentesis were analysed in relation to a range of survey variables, namely the mother's age, socioeconomic and marital status, previous pregnancy problems and parity, and concern for both her own health and that of the baby. The few statistically significant relationships which emerged are summarised in Table 4.1.

Maternal marital and socio-economic status, previous pregnancy problems, number of previous pregnancies, and concern for the health of the baby did not relate significantly to any of the above variables,

Table 4.1 Predictors of Maternal Take-up of Genetic Screening or Testing

Acceptance of either test (serum screening or amniocentesis) if offered (N = 159)

Predictor	N	Odds (95% confidence intervals)	Probability
Perceived test choice			0.000
Amniocentesis only	43	1	
Serum screening only	76	7.5 (3.2–17.4)	0.000
Serum screening or amniocentesis	40	3.9 (1.6–9.8)	0.003

Acceptance of serum screening if offered (N = 116)

Predictor	N	Odds (95% confidence intervals)	Probability
Perceived test choice			
Serum screening or amniocentesis	39	1	
Serum screening only	77	4.4 (1.8–10.5)	0.001
Concern about own health			
Yes	11	1	
No	105	4.2 (1.1–16.3)	0.04

Acceptance of amniocentesis if offered (N = 82)

Predictor	N	Odds (95% confidence intervals)	Probability
Perceived test choice			
Serum screening or amniocentesis	39	1	
Amniocentesis only	43	4.6 (1.5–14.4)	0.009
Maternal age			
<35	29	1	
35+	53	4.7 (1.3–17.0)	0.02

and were eliminated from all three logistic regression models once per-ceived choice of test was taken into account. Other studies have yielded inconsistent findings. Press and Browner (1998) also concluded that acceptance of serum screening was unrelated to maternal age, socio-economic status or parity. Marteau *et al.* (1992b) found no relation-ship between acceptance of amniocentesis and socio-economic status. In contrast, Marriott, Pelz and Kunze (1990), found, in Germany, that among women aged over 35, those of higher socio-economic status were more likely to accept prenatal diagnosis. The present findings suggest that, for those who have entered the preventative system, the main identified factor associated with their screening/testing decision is the range of available options, although older, higher risk women were more likely to accept amniocentesis. Reasons for these mostly null findings will be discussed further below.

The second part of Table 4.1 shows that women who were more concerned about their own health were less likely to accept serum screening. This finding suggests that more worried women tended not only to be treated as if they were genetically older, as shown in Chapter 3, but to act as if they were older, rejecting the less serious test option to a greater extent. (Women concerned about their own health were also more likely to accept amniocentesis, but this relationship did not attain statistical significance, perhaps because of small sample and sub-sample sizes.)

The main determinant of a woman's decision about genetic tests highlighted in Table 4.1 is not her personal characteristics but the options which she identifies as available to her. Women were more likely to accept amniocentesis if it was the only test offered, but were also more likely to end up untested. (The difference between women offered serum screening as against a choice of amniocentesis or serum screening did not approach statistical significance ($P = 0.14$), and can be dismissed as a chance finding.)

Doctors who wish to steer older, higher risk, women, aged well over 35, towards amniocentesis face the following risk management dilemma. On the one hand, if they only offer this more powerful but also more invasive test, then they will increase the proportion of higher risk women who will not accept any test. On the other hand, if they give all women a choice, then they will increase the proportion of higher risk women who opt for the less invasive, but also less accurate, alternative. This analysis is only intended to be descriptive. We do not suggest that doctors or other health professionals should try to influence pregnant women's decisions by controlling their menus of risk management choices, only that if they do so, they will encounter the above dilemma.

Finally, Table 4.1 shows that older maternal age was significantly related to acceptance of amniocentesis but not serum screening. The former finding can be readily explained in utilitarian terms. Since older women faced a higher probability of giving birth to a baby with Down's syndrome, the expected positive utility of taking the more accurate test, amniocentesis, was more likely to outweigh the negative utility arising from accepting a possibly greater risk of miscarriage.

Other studies generate a variable picture of this relationship, however. Evans *et al.* (1993) found that women of higher parity, and therefore older average age, were more likely to accept amniocentesis, a finding which matches our own. Marteau *et al.* (1992b) found no relationship between maternal age and acceptance of amniocentesis. An Australian study of women aged 37 and over (Halliday, Lumley and Watson, 1995) concluded that women undergoing their fourth or subsequent pregnancy were significantly less likely to accept amniocentesis or chorionic villus sampling than those experiencing their first, second or third. Exclusion of women aged under 37 from this study would have attenuated any relationship between maternal age/parity and rejection of amniocentesis. Moreover, no relationship between parity and take-up of the above tests was found among women who had been pregnant less than three times. The above authors explain their findings by arguing that, in the multicultural population from which their sample was drawn, women who had undergone a large number of pregnancies would be more likely to hold anti-abortion beliefs. In our own study, only a small proportion of the sample (5.2 per cent, 80) had been pregnant more than three times. In a population with a relatively low level of religious belief, high parity may not have been associated with anti-abortion attitudes. We found that age and parity were closely associated and that lower parity was significantly related to rejection of amniocentesis. However, age rather than parity was selected into the logistic regression model.

A similar relationship between older age and acceptance of serum screening might have been expected, given its negative side-effects, namely high anxiety during the period of waiting for test results and the risk of false positives. No such relationship was found, regardless of how age differences were grouped, or whether the oldest women, or those who had accepted amniocentesis were left out of the analysis. Although the null hypothesis cannot formally be accepted, we will speculate below, as to why maternal age and acceptance of serum screening may be unrelated. We will support, with qualitative data, the view that our respondents, in general, treated serum screening as a costless option, lacking drawbacks to be weighed against the risk of Down's syndrome going undetected.

Why weren't older women more likely to accept serum screening?

This section will discuss possible explanations for our tentative conclusion that willingness to accept serum screening, if offered, was unrelated to maternal age. This conclusion appears, at first sight, to suggest that women were acting irrationally, failing to take into account utilitarian considerations (Heyman, 1998, pp. 7–8). Individual views should vary. But we would anticipate a population shift towards greater uptake of serum screening at older maternal ages if women take account of their age-related probability of giving birth to a baby with Down's syndrome. Even if this relationship was attenuated by greater acceptance of amniocentesis at the oldest ages, we might expect a lower rate of acceptance of serum screening among the youngest women. The hospital policy of mainly targeting the genetic screening/testing programme at older women filtered out most of those aged under 35, and we have seen that more risk conscious, younger women were selectively offered genetic tests. Nevertheless, given the importance placed on maternal age-related risk, the lack of a relationship between maternal age and acceptance of serum screening requires explanation.

Women may have disregarded age-related risk because they decided that acceptance of serum screening was free of cost to them. Over 80 per cent accepted serum screening if it was the only test offered (see Figure 3.1). If women viewed serum screening as cost-free, then it would be worth taking, regardless of the degree of benefit obtained in terms of risk reduction. Press and Browner (1994) argued that health-care providers, attempting to reduce the prevalence of disability in the population, and pregnant women, seeking reassurance, share a common interest in believing that screening contributes to a healthy birth. But they argue that *'this optimistic faith must coexist with the more ominous themes of serious birth anomalies, selective abortion, and eugenic selection'* (p. 203). Such collusive optimism, underpinned by faith in science, makes both professionals and pregnant women reluctant to communicate openly about the adverse consequences of genetic screening. The above researchers found that 85 per cent of women aged under 36 who accepted serum screening said that they did not deliberate much before deciding, and that the most common response to the question, *'Did you think a lot before you decided to be tested?'* was *'No'* (Press and Browner, 1997, p. 984). Other studies have shown, similarly, that women who accepted serum screening did not fully understand how they might feel whilst waiting for test results and the problems arising from screening positive (Roelofson, 1993; Smith *et al.*, 1994).

A midwife, who had had more opportunity to reflect on the implications of screening/testing than most pregnant women, made both of these points.

Previously pregnant midwife: *And, as I say, sometimes they haven't thought it* [decision about screening/testing] *out as fully as they should. And they haven't had the information, and they decide on the spot. And sometimes they are devastated when they get these high levels* [of risk from serum screening]. *And then, when they come, and they are in a high risk. What to do now? Where to go?* (Jessica, midwife, aged 42, interview, post-partum, amniocentesis)

This respondent's comments suggest that women lacking her professional experience of the maternity system may choose genetic screening without appreciating the consequences, and are, therefore, not giving informed consent. One study found that, even among women who eventually terminate their pregnancy because of a genetic abnormality, 40 per cent felt that they had not fully considered the implications of accepting serum screening (White-van Mourik, 1992).

Value judgements and decision-making

As noted in the Introduction, a risk statement lumps together a synthesis of judgements about the probability of an adverse event class and about its degree of adversity. In current parlance, the terms risk and probability are often used interchangeably, so that the phrases 'risk of live births of babies with Down's syndrome' and 'probability of live births of babies with Down's syndrome' will be heard as equivalent. Juxtaposition of these alternatives brings out their difference, namely that the risk statement smuggles in an implicit value judgement about the adversity of the event which is being predicted. Having a baby with Down's syndrome may be viewed in many different ways ranging from positive acceptance to vehement rejection. These culturally and personally conditioned value judgements can be applied only to the iconic category of variable health statuses which is labelled Down's syndrome, as argued in Chapter 1. Women had to weigh up their valuation of bringing up a child with the condition against their assessment of those incommensurable consequences of prevention which they identified.

The two quotations given below illustrate the different ways in which two of these incommensurables, parenting a child with Down's syndrome and miscarriage, can be summed up.

Pregnant woman: *I just know that the risk of 1 in 200 of losing it is far less for me than having to cope with a Down's syndrome. I just*

couldn't do it. (Joan, aged 37, interview after taped hospital consultation [Bell], 11 weeks, amniocentesis)
Pregnant woman: *I get worked up more about the miscarriage than I
do about the Down's syndrome, although I definitely don't want a Down's
syndrome baby. I just, the thought of having a miscarriage and having a
healthy baby, when it is probably the only chance I'm going to get to get
pregnant, you know, it upsets me more* (Marietta, aged 39, interview after
taped hospital consultation [Laughton], 12 weeks, amniocentesis)

The second respondent's highly negative evaluation of miscarriage was
linked to its personal context, her perception that she probably would
not be able to become pregnant again. Although she eventually opted
for amniocentesis on the grounds that *'we couldn't cope with it'*, this
respondent was still *'changing my mind'* about *'such a cruel decision'*
at the time of the above interview. As noted in the Introduction, the
proposition that amniocentesis causes miscarriages has been questioned. This woman, as did many others, based her decision on the
conventional risk wisdom, variably presented (see Chapter 7), which
doctors provided.

Acceptance of Down's syndrome

A positive welcome for children with Down's syndrome cannot be
expected in a culture which places premium value on individual
achievement and physical appearance. However, some women who
rejected genetic screening/testing were prepared to at least accept such
a child, usually because they ruled out abortion. (Other women who
had ruled out abortion accepted screening for informational reasons, as
will be seen below.)

The next quotation illustrates a form of utilitarian reasoning which
derives rejection of screening from the exclusion of abortion.

Pregnant woman: *No, I didn't have anything because I couldn't. I
mean, the blood test was a means to an end. It was if you were in a high
factor you would go on for the amnio. And then, if there was something
wrong, you are doing it because you are going to abort.* (Diane, aged 38,
interview, 16 weeks, no genetic tests)

Both Edem *et al.* (1985) and Marteau *et al.* (1991) found, not surprisingly, that uptake of amniocentesis among women aged over 38 was
associated with less negative maternal attitudes towards abortion. The
above qualitative data illustrate this quantitative finding.

Women who had decisively rejected genetic screening/testing faced the problem of how to steer their way clear of this preventative system. Although, as we shall see in Chapters 6 and 7, doctors made a great effort to open up choice, women could occasionally become entangled with a system which, ultimately, was designed to abort foetuses defined as defective. The pregnant midwife quoted below, who regarded abortion as *'just killing'* emphasised this danger.

> **Pregnant midwife:** *I think that, just in view of my age, they will treat me like an old lady, you know. And once they start poking around and messing about you know, then I think . . . that's where it really gets going. So my intention would be to stay well clear.* (Jackie, midwife, aged 36, interview, 14 weeks, no genetic tests)

The next respondent cited also rejected screening/testing because she was opposed to abortion, and unwilling to accept the greater risk of miscarriage associated with amniocentesis.

> **Pregnant woman:** *I had a time with the Down's syndrome. That was horrendous . . . because of the age thing, people telling you that if you're a certain, well, over 30 there's a risk, and over 35 there is like a bigger risk and everything, you know. So we thought, 'We'll look into it'. And we'd decided that, if the baby was Down's, we would keep the baby, no question, you know, and we were both happy with that.* (Doreen, aged 38, interview, 28 weeks, no genetic tests)

This respondent viewed caring for a child with Down's syndrome as a relatively benign contingency which she felt *'happy'* about. However, lacking insider knowledge, she had found it more difficult than the last quoted respondent to stay *'well clear'* of the screening/testing system.

> **Pregnant woman:** [Hospital doctor] *just seemed to think that if I was in that age group, I had to have the test. And I said, 'Well, what is the point? Even if the test comes back that the baby's Down's, I'm not going to do anything. And, on the other hand, the baby may be healthy, and I may have a miscarriage* [from amniocentesis].' *But I couldn't get through to* [the doctor]. *A just plain headache was turning into a migraine. And* [doctor] *said, 'Well, I can't just let you go with that. You'll have to talk to the consultant.' And I thought, 'Oh God, I've got to get out of here now.'*

I said, 'I'll take the blood test then', you know, will that keep [the doctor]
*happy? But it's not very, em, it's just an indicator whether to take the other
test really isn't it?*
Interviewer: *So it wasn't for you, really, that you had it?*
Pregnant woman: *It was for* [the doctor]. (Doreen, aged 38, interview, 28 weeks, no genetic testing)

This case stood out as an untypical exception. Doctors did not generally attempt to propel women into the genetic screening/testing process
against their wishes. Their influence, if any, was exercised more gently,
as we shall see in Chapter 7. However, the above quotation does
illustrate the potential for conflict between professionals operating a risk
management system based on categorisation of a contingency as intrin-
sically adverse and those service users who do not accept this assumption. Women who would not have accepted amniocentesis on account
of the perceived risk of miscarriage could be pressured into accepting
serum screening because they regarded this test as costless.

More insidiously, women who have ruled out termination, and who
do not wish to receive advance knowledge about the genetic status of
their baby, could feel obliged to accept genetic screening out of a sense
of obligation.

Interviewer: *So, when you booked in, they asked you if you wanted the
blood test?*
Pregnant woman: *Yeah, they looked at me history, and then they said,
'Well, you are 35, so I think we'll give you the – would you like the blood
test?' They says you don't have to have it. But I think, when you are offered
something, I think you feel, well, I feel guilty, so I took it.* (Wendy, aged
35, interview, 29 weeks, serum screening)

These examples support our interpretation of the survey finding that
acceptance of serum screening, if offered, was unrelated to maternal age
or any other variable. Women tended to treat serum screening as free
of adverse consequences, and so were willing to undergo the test even
if they regarded it as pointless. However, as noted above, they, perhaps,
did not consider the impact on themselves or their families of a higher
risk result.

Coping with Down's syndrome

The above women ruled out amniocentesis and/or termination, and so
did not need to weigh up the implications of bringing up a child with

Down's syndrome, since they could not control the genetic fate of their next child. Other women, who were willing to at least entertain the idea of accepting amniocentesis and termination, concentrated on the other side of the cost/benefit equation, attempting to estimate the impact on themselves and their families of caring for a child with Down's syndrome. They mostly rejected the idea of this condition as an inherent disaster, but calibrated its adversity in terms of their own ability to cope and the degree of support they would receive from their family. Hence, their judgements were socially contextualised, whilst doctors were concerned primarily with reducing the population of children with a medically defined condition. Rothman (1988) found, similarly, that women in the USA calibrated the adversity of caring for a child with Down's syndrome in the context of their wider lives. For example, women reasoned that twin full-time careers made looking after such a child impractical, or that medical and developmental services were lacking in a rural area.

The respondent quoted below felt that, on balance, she could cope with bringing up a child with Down's syndrome.

> **Pregnant woman:** *We had different views, I must admit, because* [husband] *said he doesn't think that he could cope with a Down's baby. He couldn't cope with anything like that, he'd run a mile he would. But, em, I don't know, it's different now. I mean, maybe a few years ago, before I had* [two previous children] *I could easily have coped with a Down's . . . And if we did have a Down's baby, which I don't think we will,* [husband] *will come round. I can't see him running a mile or, you know, he's not the type.* (Patricia, interview, 24 weeks, serum screening)

The adversity of Down's syndrome was here linked to the family's capacity to cope, and was, therefore, not treated as an intrinsic quality of the condition. This capacity was, in turn, related to parental age and family responsibility. Finally, the woman's assessment of the manageability of this complex problem takes into account her husband's attitude which his wife felt able to influence so that he would 'come round'. Her confidence that her husband would not run away from the problem of caring for a child with Down's syndrome can be related to the view, expressed by a number of women, that men tend to avoid difficult issues. Although she exonerated him, this respondent implied that other husbands might not possess his sterling character. Lippman-Hand and Fraser (1979b) also found that women could reject genetic tests on the grounds of their anticipated ability to cope with a worst-case scenario involving the occurrence of the genetic abnormality in question. For women who construct an acceptable worst case, a given probability of a genetic abnormality becomes less adverse if not irrelevant. The above woman's decision to take serum screening seems discrepant with her judgement that the family could cope with caring for a child with Down's syndrome. However, she took the test to obtain *'peace of mind'*, in effect gambling on a negative, low-risk result.

The following respondent also related her coping ability to the demands placed on her by the requirement to look after other children, and decided that, on balance, she could manage.

> **Pregnant woman:** *Well, actually, the second one* [child] *was OK. I said I don't want any more tests, although I did give it more thought, that we already had one child – will we be able to cope?* (Doreen, aged 38, interview, 28 weeks, no genetic tests)

The adversity of Down's syndrome was, again, assessed in relation to overall family functioning. The next respondent quoted had unhesitatingly opted for amniocentesis because she felt unable to look after a child with the condition.

> **Interviewer:** *What was it that made you so adamant to have the amniocentesis . . . ?*
> **Previously pregnant midwife:** *I didn't really want to have a Down's syndrome baby.*
> **Interviewer:** *Right. And why was that?*
> **Previously pregnant midwife:** *Knowing what kind of responsibility that would put on us. And, I suppose, the fact, I don't know whether my decision would have been any different if I had been younger. I probably wouldn't have had the opportunity had I been younger, but whether it would have made me feel different I don't know. But the fact that I was almost 40 when I had* [previous child], *so to have a Down's syndrome would have been very difficult to bring up, and I just didn't want to do it I suppose. And long-term prospects for the child, because of my age.* (Jessica, midwife, aged 42, interview, post-partum, amniocentesis)

This woman explained her inability to cope in terms of her present age, and of anticipated future problems, which might include parental death whilst the child was still a young adult. Although all parents of a possible Down's syndrome child face this problem, it may loom larger for those who have accepted that they have passed into middle age. This response illustrates the concepts of vital and lifespan age, discussed in Chapter 2.

The confidence of the woman quoted previously that her husband would ultimately support her sustained her decision to rule out termination. In contrast, this last respondent's feeling that her husband would evade difficult problems may have contributed to her clear rejection of a future which involved bringing up a Down's syndrome child.

> **Interviewer:** *What was the main thing that you worried about with your age, when you say that your risk . . . ?*
> **Previously pregnant woman:** *It's abnormalities . . .*
> **Interviewer:** *Was your husband the same was he . . . ?*
> **Previously pregnant woman:** *No. He didn't think of that aspect, he would rather not think.* (Jessica, midwife, aged 42, interview, postpartum, amniocentesis)

The next respondent also linked the adversity of caring for a child with Down's syndrome to problems in coping, and in turn associated such problems with her own age. As noted in Chapter 2, this view was predicated on the assumption that growing older brings about a decline in maternal coping capacity.

> **Pregnant woman:** *You know, I'm not a very patient person to start with. If I had one of them, I don't, I definitely couldn't have coped. I mean, saying that, when I had [older child] I thought, well, if it's like that I would bring it up, and cope with her like. So it must be really me age, because I wouldn't have minded if, you know, she was like that.* (Angela, aged 38, interview, 22 weeks, serum screening)

This respondent accounted for her projected inability to cope in terms of the combination of an enduring temperamental limitation, not being 'patient', and an age-related reduction in resilience. Her judgement was influenced by a concrete experience of the demanding nature of another child with Down's syndrome.

> **Interviewer:** *Is that* [Down's syndrome] *the main concern?*
> **Pregnant woman:** *Aha . . . My cousin's got one. She's got a little boy, and I don't know how she copes with him. He's six now, but on the go constantly, even during the night. And I say I definitely couldn't cope with one of them.* (Angela, aged 38, interview, 22 weeks, serum screening)

Her reasoning was based on induction from a single case, and predicated on the assumption that this boy's hyperactivity was both caused by and characteristic of Down's syndrome.

Rejection of Down's syndrome

The women quoted above judged the adversity of this event in relation to their social circumstances and coping ability. Others rejected outright the idea of becoming the parent of a child with Down's syndrome.

> **Woman anticipating pregnancy:** *The way I feel at the moment, I would go straight for the amnio. I really want to talk to somebody more about it. The knowledge I have got so far is that the blood test can only tell me whether I am at high risk or low risk. It can't tell me definitely, and I have got this phobia about Down's syndrome . . . If the amnio can tell me more, I would want to go for that, even though I am aware of the risk that I may lose the baby. I don't know if that is a really selfish thing.* (Yvonne, aged 35, interview, not pregnant, intending to choose amniocentesis)

Her '*phobia*' about Down's syndrome tipped the balance for this woman towards amniocentesis at a maternal age which doctors at our hospital research site considered marginal even for serum screening. The quotation illustrates particularly clearly the utilitarian calculations behind many women's decisions. Both the value and the probability of the event class on which preventative attention is focused are taken into account, and a high degree of negativity counterbalances a relatively low probability of an adverse event. This highly negative assessment, in turn, substantially raised this woman's threshold of acceptability for the probability of miscarriage resulting from amniocentesis.

> **Woman anticipating pregnancy:** *I do want to know more information about how risky the amnio is, and what the actual statistics are. If it was a 50 per cent chance I could miscarry I might think twice about it.* (Yvonne, aged 35, interview, not pregnant, intending to choose amniocentesis)

Probability estimation and decision-making

Risk calculations entail combining value and probabilistic judgements about selected consequences over a time frame which the person making the calculation must specify (see the Introduction). We will now discuss in some detail the ways in which women understood probabilistic reasoning, and drew upon their understanding in their decision-making about genetic screening/testing for Down's syndrome. We will first explore their understanding of the probability heuristic, the concept of which was outlined in the Introduction, and then consider women's personal probabilistic reasoning.

The probability heuristic

Epidemiological risk analysis is based on unreflexive employment of the probability heuristic (Heyman, Henriksen and Maughan, 1998), as argued in the Introduction. Use of this heuristic entails inductive estimation of the rates of a condition in aggregated groups, and assignment of these rates to new individuals who meet the criteria for group membership. Categorisation of probabilistic knowledge as heuristic undermines the official line which pits scientific rationality, taken for granted as unproblematic, against lay simplification. We do not seek to assign equivalent status to lay and scientific reasoning about probability, but to argue that the former entail a simplification of a simplification.

As with any other heuristic, for example availability, discussed below, the usefulness of the probability heuristic can be assessed in terms of its power to make manageable complexity which the heuristic user otherwise could not handle with a given stock of knowledge. But this gain must be offset against the inevitable distortions which result from simplification. Ideally, doctors should be able to specify individual outcomes with perfect accuracy. Women who wish to know whether their baby has chromosomal abnormalities, but who are not prepared to buy near certainty by accepting the risks associated with diagnostic tests, have to rely on inductive, probabilistic knowledge. This knowledge is based on a simplifying fiction which requires acceptance of the ecological fallacy that individuals carry with them a similar share of the aggregates on which induction is based. Ironically, this fallacy lies at the heart of epidemiological risk analysis.

Acceptance of the probability heuristic gives rise to three related types of problem for professionals who claim risk expertise, and for pregnant women who are required to base a vital personal decision on this knowledge. We will discuss below the problems of limited predictive power, multiple probabilities of the same event, and changing probabilities of the same event.

Limited predictive power

Pregnant women did not always understand the inductively estimated aggregate rates on which the probability heuristic is based.

> **Pregnant woman:** *There was a 1 per cent risk of amniocentesis and miscarriage, but* [hospital doctor] *wouldn't say what the percentage was. I mean, is it 1 per cent in 100, 1 per cent in a thousand or . . . ?* [The doctor] *didn't tell me that.* (Marietta, aged 39, interview after hospital consultation [Laughton], 12 weeks, amniocentesis)

As pregnant women themselves sometimes point out, the probability heuristic, even when properly explained and understood, cannot tell women within a risk category whether they personally will or will not encounter the event in question. Women are informed about the proportion of a defined category, to which they have been assigned, who will experience a given contingency. But they cannot be told which emergent sub-category, of those who do and do not experience the contingency, they will eventually belong to. This is the question which women, concerned about their own individual fates, not those of aggregates, want answered. They may use its unanswerability to subvert the probability heuristic itself.

> **Pregnant midwife:** *But, there again, I could have a nice healthy baby. I don't need it* [genetic screening/testing]. *I could have had a Down's syndrome baby at 26.* (Shirley, midwife, aged 34, interview, 20 weeks, no genetic tests)

Lippman-Hand and Fraser (1979a) found that some of their counsellees expressed similar reservations about the limitations of rate-based prognostication. The doctor quoted next acknowledged this limitation in a way which maintained the probability heuristic.

> **Doctor:** *So, firstly, the thing about Down's Syndrome is to say that any woman who is pregnant can have a baby with Down's Syndrome. All women have a risk. If you are 19 you have a risk. If you are 49 you have a risk. It's just that, in relation to your age, the risk increases.* (Susan, aged 35, hospital consultation [Gould], 15 weeks, serum screening)

The above formulation makes probability a property of women, rather than of limited knowledge. If they took a perfectly accurate test, then none of those tested would *'have a risk'*, since they would know with certainty that their baby either had, or did not have, Down's syndrome. Doctors adopted the same natural attitude towards risk as is found in the wider culture, projecting it onto the world as an attribute of events. This stance obscures the epistemological status of empirically derived probabilities as descriptions of limited inductive knowledge, and therefore relative to the observer.

The following instructive quotation conveys a woman's sense of resentment at being classified as a member of a risk category, rather than as a unique individual.

Pregnant woman: *You don't want to be told like, you want to be told that there's a risk, but you don't want to be quoted numbers. I felt that that was, like, a bit impersonal, you know, to be told about statistics and that, and things like that . . . I just wanted to know what, what could be done and what couldn't be done, you know.* (Hilary, aged 40, interview, 23 weeks, amniocentesis)

This woman's description of risk statistics as *'impersonal'* neatly points up the simplification inherent in the probability heuristic, namely that properties of a category are attributed to the individuals within it.

Multiple probabilities of the same event

The probabilities which are assigned to individuals through the probability heuristic will depend upon the definition of risk categories. It follows, apparently paradoxically, that the same individual may have more than one probability of experiencing the same event. This paradox dissolves if the heuristic status of the fiction that aggregate statistics can be applied to individuals is taken into account.

The doctor quoted below, unusually, undermined the facticity of probabilistic induction by demonstrating that the same event could have more than one chance of occurring.

Doctor: *If you think of it in easier numbers, we deliver about 4000 . . . babies a year here. And the overall incidence of Down's Syndrome is about 1 in 500 pregnancies, which would mean that we deliver, if we didn't do these tests, 5 or 6 abnormal babies per year.* (Marietta, aged 39, hospital consultation [Laughton], 10 weeks, amniocentesis)

This way of thinking does not provide merely *'easier numbers'*, but a different probability estimate from those related to maternal age. An aggregate risk of 1 in 500 for all women can be broken down into higher and lower risks for older and younger women, and each age-related category further disaggregated in terms of screening results and other predictors. A woman could be told that she faces either of these probabilities, depending upon the category or sub-category into which she is placed. (The doctor should have referred to eight or nine abnormal babies, given the cited figures.) A follow-up interview, undertaken after the hospital consultation but before she had been tested, showed that this woman had registered both of these probabilities. Her maternal age-related risk *'depressed'* her.

> **Pregnant woman:** *Well* [the doctor] *used all these percentages, you know, and that, and you just don't look at it from that sort of point of view, you know. You think, well, just because you are 39 why should you have an abnormal baby . . . I came out depressed, went in quite chirpy came out depressed.*
> **Interviewer:** *Can you remember the percentages, can you remember what your statistics were?*
> **Pregnant woman:** *It was 120 to 1? 1 in every 120, the women my age who have Down's Syndrome, is that right?* (Marietta, aged 39, interview after taped hospital consultation [Laughton], 12 weeks, amniocentesis)

But this woman consoled herself by thinking about the alternative, smaller probability she had been offered, recalling the lowest of the range of figures which the doctor had mentioned.

> **Pregnant woman:** *That sort of, like, cheers me up, when* [the doctor] *said I was 1 in 4200, I think, or 4500 or something . . . , and only five of them were Down's Syndrome.* (Marietta, aged 39, interview after taped hospital consultation [Laughton], 12 weeks, amniocentesis)

Exposure to these two probabilities, both valid in their own terms, may have contributed to this woman's intense indecision, expressed in the above interview, about whether to select serum screening or amniocentesis.

Changing the probability of the same event

The third consequence of using the probability heuristic follows from heuristic acceptance of the ecological fallacy that aggregate properties of a category can be assigned to individual members. Probabilities can be changed merely through obtaining additional information which enables a risk category to be further subdivided. Each of the resulting sub-categories will have its own aggregate properties which will differ from those of the parent category providing that the newly introduced risk indicator is associated with the adverse event which is being predicted. The quotation below, from an interview with a pregnant midwife who had rejected genetic screening/testing for herself, discusses another woman's perception that learning the results of a screening test would change her probability of giving birth to a baby with Down's syndrome.

Pregnant midwife: *One woman who is 38, and she said that she simply didn't want screening, but felt she had to have it, not from here, but from society, because, she said, because she was 38. She just couldn't face her work mates. She couldn't face anybody with a Down's syndrome child because they would know she would have been offered screening. So then, if she had a Down's syndrome child, well, it would be her fault that she had had a Down's syndrome child. Whereas, if she had been 26, everybody would be kind of, 'Oh, that is bad luck.'* (Shirley, midwife, aged 34, interview, 20 weeks, no genetic tests)

In effect, this woman had realised, according to her midwife, that the availability of screening gave her the power to control her probability of having a baby with Down's syndrome. If she decided not to undergo a screening test, she would leave herself in the undifferentiated category of women whose chance of this event was defined by its rate in their age group. If she took the test, she would be assigned to a category with either a higher or a lower probability of this contingency, but could not know in advance which sub-category she would end up in. The quotation illustrates particularly clearly the role of risk as a forensic resource (Douglas, 1990) in risk-oriented societies. Individuals in such societies are obliged to attempt to prevent high, but not low, risks as conventionally defined. The woman whose views the above midwife reported felt that a Down's birth to a woman aged 26 would be accepted as bad luck, whilst a woman aged 39 would be deemed irresponsible for not refining her risk estimate. The social processes through which the dividing line between high and low risk is set in a particular context remain unexamined in the background.

Because of the accuracy of amniocentesis, women who chose this test could change their probability of giving birth to a baby with Down's syndrome to almost 1 or 0, although, again, they could not know in advance which outcome would result, and had to accept a possible risk of miscarriage in order to banish uncertainty. The following insightful quotation, from an interview with another pregnant midwife, illustrates the way in which a woman could control her own probability of a future event through her screening/testing decisions.

> **Pregnant midwife:** *I didn't want to have the, em, I could have had the amnio, because I didn't want to be placed in a position of having to decide about a termination, because I knew I wouldn't want one. But I thought, once you know for a fact that you have a Down's syndrome child, would that change you? Would you then want to have a termination because you would feel pressure . . . from other people.* (Jackie, midwife, aged 36, interview, 14 weeks, no genetic tests)

Women could decide not to be categorised into sub-groups with lower and higher aggregate probabilities of giving birth to a baby with Down's syndrome, refusing genetic tests. But they could not escape the onus of having made this decision. A woman who declines genetic screening and testing and gives birth to a baby with Down's syndrome must accept that she chose not to take preventative action. Hence, women's freedom to manage their own futures was constrained by the mere availability of the genetic screening/testing system (Green, Statham and Snowdon, 1992). They could not choose not to make a choice once genetic screening or testing had been offered. The provision of this preventative system forms part of a wider societal process of individualisation (Beck, 1992; Beck-Gernsheim, 1996), in which individual responsibility for personal futures is expanding inexorably.

Personal probability assessment

Older women who regarded Down's syndrome as an adverse event did not necessarily assess themselves as facing a high probability of the condition. Women of any age can carry a baby with Down's syndrome. The hospital policy of not offering tests to younger women unless they had a family history of the condition implicitly communicated to these younger women that their risk could be discounted. We will now contrast the views of older women who did and did not see themselves as at risk, and then explore their views of the divide, if any, between high and low risk.

Acceptance of maternal age as an indicator of high risk

Many older women took it for granted that they were at high risk of having a baby with genetic abnormalities. They experienced considerable anxiety and even guilt in consequence. The following respondent weighed up both her age and her reproductive history, concluding that she would probably have a child with a genetic abnormality.

> **Interviewer:** *Did you feel your risks had increased from* [previous child]. *Were you conscious of that or . . . ?*
> **Previously pregnant midwife:** *Well obviously, you know, the risks increase, but . . . I suppose the same thing came into play with* [previous child] *really, the fact that I had had an* [spontaneous] *abortion before . . . meant, most likely, that I would have a child with some kind of a chromosomal abnormality.* (Jessica, midwife, aged 42, interview, post-partum, amniocentesis)

Because of this assessment of her risk, the above respondent had *'made certain that I had an amniocentesis'*, even though she remained un-decided about going through with a termination in the event of a positive result. This vivid depiction of risk concern illustrates the quan-titative finding (Marteau *et al.*, 1991) that women are more likely to accept amniocentesis if they assess their personal probability of giving birth to a baby with Down's syndrome as high, regardless of their 'actual', that is, maternal age-related, risk.

However, her previous miscarriage could have occurred for many reasons, and provided only a weak indicator of additional risk. At the age of 42, her maternal age-related risk of giving birth to a baby with Down's syndrome would have been estimated as about 1:60. Although 'high' at the population level, and in comparison with younger women, such a probability did not make a Down's syndrome birth *'most likely'*. This confusion arose in a medical context which defined maternal age over 40 as a serious health problem.

Another older woman felt guilty about, as she saw it, putting her baby at unacceptable risk.

> **Pregnant woman:** *I thought because I've made a decision to get preg-nant at this age, I've put the baby at risk.* (Beatrice, aged 40, interview, 26 weeks, amniocentesis)

Not surprisingly, given her perception of the seriousness of the genetic risk which she faced, this woman had no hesitation about opting for amniocentesis. However, she may not have appreciated that, according to the table which doctors used when advising women about genetic risks, she faced an age-related probability of about 1:110 of giving birth to a baby with Down's syndrome.

The following example is unusual in two respects, but instructive. Firstly, the respondent, who had decided on amniocentesis and termination if necessary, was concerned that the risks facing older women might be underestimated, rather than exaggerated. Secondly, her concern had been triggered by an incident involving exposure of the gambler's fallacy. An older friend had given birth to two disabled children in sequence, following the birth of a normal child.

> **Pregnant woman:** *And she* [older friend] *wanted reassurance that this baby wasn't going to be handicapped. And then it was a case of you never have two handicapped together* [second oldest and expected child]. *And so* [friend] *was conned* [whilst in hospital] *into thinking she couldn't have* [another handicapped child]. (Lesley, aged 37, interview, 26 weeks, amniocentesis)

The gambler fallacy is based on the assumption that an event which is expected to occur with a regular frequency but in an irregular order, and which has occurred in a regular sequence, for example a series of reds on the roulette wheel, will be unlikely to recur. The above respondent believed that, in the case of her friend, hospital staff had committed this fallacy, and so provided false reassurance. Epidemiologically, the birth of a child with disabilities would, if anything, lead to a prediction of increased risk of abnormalities in subsequent children. Her acceptance of amniocentesis at a relatively young age may have been triggered by the ensuing mistrust which she experienced. Such examples demonstrate that decisions about health risks must be understood in relation to individuals' wider frameworks of understanding.

Another respondent who accepted that she was at risk reasoned that the occurrence of Down's syndrome births involving younger women demonstrated the even greater risk faced by older women.

> **Pregnant woman:** *That* [Down's syndrome]*'s my main concern.*
> **Interviewer:** *Why is that?*
> **Pregnant woman:** *Just because of my age, and just because people say it happens when you are that age. And I know girls younger than me that have Down's babies, or that have had Down's babies. I know a girl 23 that had a Down's baby.* (Patricia, aged 37, interview, 24 weeks, serum screening)

This line of reasoning excludes consideration of the much larger denominator for births to younger than to older women, and so elevates the greater level of risk to the latter. It involves use of the availability heuristic (Tversky and Kahneman, 1973), probabilistic generalisation from individually known cases. More commonly, as will be seen in the next section, older respondents cited examples of younger women giving birth to babies with Down's syndrome in order to challenge the system of knowledge which categorised them as facing a higher risk of this outcome.

Although our discussion of age-related risks has focused on the decisions of older women, younger respondents did not dismiss these concerns as irrelevant to themselves. At the extreme, the respondent quoted below challenged the moral integrity of older parents who, in her view, placed the unborn child at unacceptable risk through late pregnancy.

> **Interviewer:** *What do you think about the women who are older, who have babies in their 30s or later?*
>
> **Pregnant woman:** *I think, if you want a baby you shouldn't think about you, but about the bairn, because you have got more chance of having a disabled baby, the older you are . . .*
>
> **Interviewer:** *Do you think they should have the testing to see if the child is disabled?*
>
> **Pregnant woman:** *Yes, but then the child is already inside of them. I would hate to be put in that position, and I am pleased I am having two healthy babies.* (Caroline, aged 18, interview, 20 weeks, no genetic tests)

This view, although unusually harsh, defined a moral order, predicated upon a risk appraisal, which castigates older parents who choose to accept a higher probability of genetic abnormalities for their child. The youngest pregnant women often feel vulnerable to criticism for their own pregnancy timing. A highly critical stance towards the oldest group may provide a means of bolstering the legitimacy of their own position (Aarvold, 1998).

Rejection of maternal age as an indicator of high risk

Other older women did not accept the categorisation of themselves as high risk cases, and could support their position in two ways. Firstly, they could point to the in-built limitation of the probability heuristic, discussed above, namely that most high risk cases would not experience the predicted negative event, whilst some individuals in the low risk group would do so. Secondly, they could define their maternal age-related probability of giving birth to a baby with Down's syndrome as a low risk.

The woman quoted below derived *'comfort'* from her knowledge of older women who had borne healthy babies, and cited the case of a baby with Down's syndrome born to a much younger mother.

> **Pregnant woman:** *My husband knows someone who was only in his early 40s now, and he's got a Down's syndrome boy, and he's in his 20s. And both him and his wife were in their early 20s when they had him. And I think, well, it can happen at that age, it can happen any time.* (Diane, aged 38, interview, 16 weeks, no genetic tests)

Lippman (1999) also found, in her qualitative study, that some older women used this argument to challenge the medical categorisation of them as at higher risk. Women who reasoned in this way, rejecting both the power and the limitations of the average, could not avoid confronting the unpredictability of genetic events. The resulting heightened feelings of uncertainty could themselves generate anxiety, as reported by the last woman quoted.

The next respondent, similarly, used cases of health problems experienced by the offspring of young, fit parents, and of their absence in the children of older parents, to undermine the status of parental age as a risk indicator. This example also illustrates the use of generalisation from experience or from other health problem to maternal age-related genetic risk.

> **Interviewer:** *Have you had any particular worries?*
> **Pregnant woman:** *Not particular ones . . . I have had two aunts who have had children very late, well into their forties, and the kids are my age, and most of them were fine . . . The person who's had the worst problems is a friend of mine . . . He [child] had, the arteries and veins in his heart were all wrong, and he ended up having major heart surgery when he was six weeks old. And they've had major trauma with him. And yet, to look at them, they were two people who did everything right. They were dead fit.* (Ann, aged 34, interview, 20 weeks, no genetic tests)

The example which she cited in order to undermine the categorisation of herself as a high risk case did not involve a parental age-related chromosomal abnormality. Her reasoning relied both on the availability heuristic and on generalisation from conditions with a prevalence unrelated to maternal age.

According to the midwife quoted below, one woman had cited the normal outcome of her own previous pregnancy as evidence that she did not need to worry about Down's syndrome.

Previously pregnant midwife: *One of my really intelligent girls . . . had an amnio with* [daughter from previous pregnancy], *and then was pregnant with this one two years on. And I said to her, 'Have you thought, are you going to have an amnio again?'. She is 38 to 40. And she said, 'Oh no, my last one was fine.' And I said, 'Well, that is not a written guarantee, that because one amnio is fine that this one is fine', you know, trying to explain the genetics. And I said, 'This is a totally different baby.' And she said, 'Oh no my last one was fine, so this will be fine.' And she just totally dealt with, wouldn't talk about it any further. So, whether that was her way of coping?* (Tina, midwife, aged 37, interview, post-partum, serum screening)

The sense of safety of the woman referred to, again depended upon use of the availability heuristic (Tversky and Kahneman, 1973). However, this simplification was itself applied to a simplifying device, the probability heuristic. Professionals were hampered in their rebuttals of propositions based on the availability heuristic by the limitation inherent in their own prognostic knowledge, namely, as already noted, that it was derived from populations, but applied to individuals.

A second way in which older pregnant women could challenge the characterisation of them as high risk cases involved accepting the official maternal age-related probability, but categorising it as low.

Pregnant woman: *Let's see, how I can put this, I think, I know, the risks are very slight anyway. And I would rather just go ahead with the pregnancy than have a termination.* (Patricia, aged 37, interview, 24 weeks, serum screening)

Her classification of the probability of this event as *'slight'* meant that it would have little negative utility (expectation times value) for her even if she viewed Down's syndrome as a highly negative event. This perspective should be contrasted with that of Jessica, quoted above, who believed that *'most likely'* she was carrying a baby with chromosomal abnormalities. Admittedly, Jessica, at 42, faced a higher risk of such problems. Nevertheless, this sharp contrast illustrates the impact of qualitative interpretation on understanding of quantitative probabilities. A given numerical probability can be categorised as high or low, depending upon where the line between these two states is drawn. Ironically, the age-related probability of a woman aged 37 giving birth to a baby with Down's Syndrome, 1:240, would be regarded as low if it was generated by serum screening. The Northern Genetics Service used a probability of 1:200 as the cut-off for recommending amniocentesis after serum screening, but encouraged women whose age-related probability of bearing a child with Down's Syndrome was below this level to consider genetic screening or testing.

The respondent quoted below, aged 36, also defined herself as being at low risk. She strengthened her case with an argument which statisticians would not endorse.

Pregnant midwife: *I found it* [statistics given at hospital consultation] *quite encouraging because I have a 1 in 311 chance, which meant that 310 people had to walk through that door before I would end up with a Down's syndrome child. And then, I mean, I asked, interestingly enough, I asked* [the doctor] *about this point, but* [the doctor] *hadn't taken it on board, and wasn't happy I raised* [it] *. . . I mean those figures are based on average childbearing. They don't take into account that less women have babies at my age, and, therefore, what figures you have are going to be unnaturally inflated, which, in my opinion, decreases my risk.* (Jackie, midwife, aged 36, interview, 14 weeks, no genetic tests)

Rapp (1988, p. 188) noted that American, middle-class pregnant women often *'fight with numbers'* by developing idiosyncratic interpretations of probabilistic reasoning. However, the above was the only such battle identified in our data. Perhaps women brought up in a health culture which centres around the British NHS are less willing to question the knowledge base which underpins their categorisation as at high risk. Her account violates probabilistic principles in two ways. It assumes that an event which occurs with a regular frequency also occurs in a regular sequence (the gambler's fallacy). And it confuses the size of the denominator in a probability estimate with the ratio between the numerator and the denominator. Her reasoning underpinned this woman's decision not to undergo genetic tests.

Maternal age as a binary risk marker

The operation of a preventative system with selective entry, as at our hospital research site, requires the specification and application of criteria which define who should and should not be invited to join the system. Such binary decision-making divides a continuous indicator

such as maternal age into two discrete categories. The resulting boundary may then be legitimated as marking a dividing line between high
and low risk cases. Acceptance of the categorisation of older women as
being at higher risk and of the facticity of this binary divide were closely
associated.

> **Pregnant woman:** *Well there is the magic age of 35 in* [other Euro-
> pean country]. *When you are pregnant at 35 you have to go in for special
> tests to find out whether the kid is normal or not, and, yeah, so I assume
> that's when the critical age starts.* (Kate, aged 32, interview, 20 weeks,
> no genetic tests)

Two interviewed women saw the dividing line between higher and lower
risk at around 35 as having magical properties. They must have assumed
that transition to the group needing tests resulted from a qualitative but
mysterious biological shift. Other, more sceptical women adopted a social
constructionist approach to this divide, as we shall show below. A woman ·
quoted at the end of this section, also described the supposed transition
as magical, but only for debunking purposes.

Women who believed in an age barrier beyond which risks became
unacceptable located this barrier at different temporal points. Our survey
and qualitative data (Henriksen and Heyman, 1998) suggest that most,
but not all, women raised the age ceiling sufficiently to be able to locate
themselves in the safe category. The next respondent quoted, aged 38,
had moved the boundary for acceptable risk up to the age of 40.

> **Interviewer:** *At what age do you think that you would feel concerned
> about being pregnant?*
> **Pregnant woman:** *Forty, I think. If you are over 40, I think you are at
> risk, the baby and yourself, aren't you? 'Cos 40's dead old, you know.*
> (Angela, aged 38, interview, 22 weeks, serum screening)

Elevation of the presumed risk boundary marker may have contributed
to this woman's decision to opt for serum screening rather than amniocentesis at a relatively 'old' age. The next quoted respondent, unusually, located herself on the wrong side of the risk boundary, and,
therefore, accepted amniocentesis.

> **Pregnant woman:** *Yes, I suppose, probably from about 36, 37, I
> thought it's a bit old now to have children because all the risks obviously
> increase as you get older.*

Interviewer: *Yes. What was the main thing that you were worried about with your age? . . .*
Pregnant woman: *It's abnormalities.* (Hilary, aged 40, interview, 23 weeks, amniocentesis)

This anomalous case contrasts with those much more common ones where older women managed to avoid defining themselves as being at high risk of genetic abnormalities, despite the messages implicit in screening programmes. The tendency to see only pregnant women older than themselves as too advanced in years to have a baby was found even among respondents aged 40 and over. Of nine out of ten women in this age group who answered the appropriate survey questions, three believed that a woman would never be too old to have a baby, whilst the other six cited age barriers which were 3–5 years above their own age. Hence, most women managed to avoid defining themselves as at unacceptably high risk. The concern of the last woman quoted may have been triggered by her husband's risk consciousness.

Interviewer: *Do you have any concerns for your own health at all with your pregnancy and delivery? . . .*
Pregnant woman: *No, me husband has . . .* [Husband] *was very, more so with us being asthmatic, and me age again. He was very, like, concerned about em, how it would be throughout the pregnancy, and after the baby was born, and that, you know, health-wise.* (Hilary, aged 40, interview, 23 weeks, amniocentesis)

Other women questioned the use of a temporal dividing line to determine eligibility for screening/testing. Some appeared no more than mildly perplexed about why women should suddenly shift from a low to a high risk category as they aged gradually. The respondent quoted below, also a midwife, had given birth to her first baby at the age of 33, and the second when she was 35. The births were thus separated by the most common dividing line used to differentiate 'high' and 'low' risk pregnances.

Previously pregnant midwife: *It's funny, isn't it, because you think, that age gap, 35, well why should I be different now? . . . And, as I say, when I was 33 I was a little bit concerned. But they didn't ask for any screening at that time.* (Jan, midwife, aged 35, interview, post-partum, serum screening)

Although the next quoted respondent had accepted serum screening out of politeness, despite ruling out amniocentesis and termination, she summarily rejected the idea of a maternal risk/age barrier.

> **Pregnant woman:** *But I think it's the 36 barriers that some people say.*
> **Interviewer:** *Do you feel that?*
> **Pregnant woman:** *Nah, it's just what it's made out to be, isn't it?* (Wendy, aged 35, interview, 29 weeks, serum screening)

This respondent's blunt rejection of the idea of a natural age barrier, beyond which pregnancy becomes dangerous, was supported by a micro-social calibration of time, since she viewed her pregnancy as not late relative to those of her immediate circle of friends. The quotation illustrates the way in which different normative time velocities, the theme of Chapter 2, could impinge upon women's understanding of age-related risks.

The next respondent referred to a magical transition, as did the woman quoted at the beginning of this section, but only to dismiss the magic as a conjuring trick.

> **Pregnant midwife:** *It is difficult to say it, but we do categorise people, we do, especially in the medical terms, you would say. Where they got the 35 from I don't know, especially when there are a lot of women having babies older and older nowadays. But this magical 35 has appeared. And if you are 35, then you are at risk. If you are approaching 35, then you are in a grey area, and don't know where you are.* (Shirley, midwife, aged 34, interview, 20 weeks, no genetic tests)

Her citation of the borderline above the age of 35 undermined the division of women into discrete, age-related risk categories. Our final quotation on this topic offers a purely pragmatic, organisational justification for distinguishing high risk cases meriting intervention from low risk cases which do not.

> **Pregnant woman:** *The only thing that makes me think is, why is amnio only offered to 35 year olds and over, because, it's just like breast screening, isn't it, over 50 year, 'cos you can get breast cancer when you are younger than 50 can't you? I suppose they've got to draw the line somewhere, yeah.* (Patricia, aged 37, interview, 24 weeks, serum screening)

However, if this pragmatic distinction is projected onto the phenomenon in question, then gradually increasing risks will be perceived as subject to qualitative shifts. Women may even bring forward their family planning, as suggested by Wendy, quoted above, in order to beat a 'magical', but mythical deadline.

5
Women's Decisions about Genetic Tests II: Time Management and Outcomes

Introduction

This chapter will complete our exploration of the genetic screening/ testing decisions made by pregnant women at our hospital research site. It will, firstly, discuss the ways in which women took account of the temporal dimension of risk, making variable allowance for differences in the timing of perceived consequences such as amniocentesis-induced miscarriage, termination and care for a child with Down's syndrome. Secondly, the chapter will consider genetic test outcomes, with respect to both the overall performance of the hospital genetic screening/testing system and the impact of genetic test results on pregnant women.

Time management

We have considered, in Chapter 2, the multidimensional calculations through which women gauged the timing of parenthood as too early, too late or on-time. They also had to weigh up the short and long-term implications of various courses of genetic action. Health professionals could afford to adopt a longer time frame. For pregnant women, their immediate futures, and the associated risks, loomed large, sometimes pushing more distant prospects into the background. Quantitative risk assessors discount time at the inflation-adjusted real rate of return in financial markets (Viscusi, 1992, p. 55). Such heuristics may provide a crude guide for large-scale risk management, but they fail to do justice to the complexities of real decision-making.

Some concerns seem timeless, for example, absolute rejection of abortion. Some are associated with the immediate process of the pregnancy, and others with events in the relatively far future, for instance, the anticipated burden of care for an adult with Down's syndrome. Consideration of consequences spread over different time-frames could incline women either towards or away from genetic screening/testing. We will focus below primarily on the temporal thinking of women who opted for amniocentesis or rejected both screening and testing, since, as we have seen, women often accepted serum screening without considering the consequences. We will first explore the impact of anticipated, shorter-term negative consequences of test acceptance. This time-frame will be contrasted with that of women who had decided to abort a baby with Down's syndrome if a genetic abnormality was discovered, and who focused on longer-term contingencies. However, we shall see that these two time-frames, encompassing the pregnancy itself as against the adulthood of a child with Down's syndrome, cannot be totally separated because consequences, for example emotional trauma, could ripple out causally into the more distant future. Finally, we will illustrate the additional complication which arose, for some women, from uncertainty about their own future intentions, particularly about whether they could actually go through with an abortion in the hypothetical circumstance that a genetic abnormality was discovered.

Short-term concerns should not be dismissed as inherently less rational than those involving the more distant future. Risk management almost always entails striking a balance between qualitatively distinct considerations which operate on different time-scales. Western culture privileges the middle-term personal biography of individuals over both the immediate present and the historical future.

Shorter-term considerations

Shorter-term considerations, centred around the pregnancy itself, could incline women to accept or reject genetic screening/testing for various reasons, outlined below.

Body violation

A few women rejected amniocentesis on account of the invasive nature of the procedure. The following quotation provides a particularly vivid example.

> **Interviewer:** *You said before about the spina bifida. Have you thought about other tests at all, like amniocentesis, or do you not know much about other tests?*

Pregnant woman: *No, not, er, I wouldn't like that one. That's where they go through the belly button, isn't it? I wouldn't like that. I keep thinking they might burst the bag or something.* (Samantha, aged 25, interview, no genetic tests)

Even if not anatomically correct, and merely hypothetical, given her age, this respondent's concern derived from her sense that surgical procedures would invasively violate her body. As always in qualitative risk analysis, we need to understand a person's preventative behaviour in terms of the risks which they perceive, not in relation to those which an external agency defines as real.

Late termination

Some women rejected genetic screening/testing on the grounds that prevention of the birth of a baby with Down's syndrome would require a late abortion.

Pregnant midwife: *It never occurred to me to have one* [genetic test] *because, it's a personal feeling, . . . If it turns out bad, what are you going to do about it? And are you prepared to do that? . . . Immediately I thought, 'Well, you're going to be doing really late terminations, in some instances.'* (Sharon, midwife, aged 31, interview, 36 weeks, no genetic tests)

Another pregnant midwife weighed up the immediate trauma of amniocentesis-induced miscarriage or termination against the future beyond her pregnancy, discounting the latter.

Pregnant midwife: *If there is a problem, would I want to put the baby at risk with amniocentesis or an abortion? Could I do that? I don't think, personally, I could. And, that way, I probably wouldn't have screening done. The consequences, I'm going to be left with, fair enough.* (Shirley, midwife, aged 34, interview, 20 weeks, no genetic tests)

Both of the above quotations were given by midwives with professional experience of the genetic screening/testing system. Most women who opted for amniocentesis did not realise what a late termination would entail. Discovery could cause considerable distress.

Pregnant woman: *And I'd also found out that you had to go through the labour* [for a termination]. *That was really, really scary, 'cos I* *never knew that at the very beginning. It wasn't until mid-flow that it sort of slipped out of somebody's mouth . . . Well that really, really panicked me.*

Interviewer: *Did you not know that 'til after you had the amniocentesis?*

Pregnant woman: *It was after the amnio.* (Lesley, aged 37, interview, 26 weeks, amniocentesis)

The above respondent had obtained crucial information, given casually, only through her own questioning. Having opted for amniocentesis without this information, she found herself engaged in a process from which she could not easily extricate herself. She might have decided to eschew genetic screening/testing if she had known that late termination would require a full labour.

Use of dilation and evacuation techniques under general anaesthetic may avoid the trauma of undergoing labour to deliver an aborted baby (Black, 1994). However, this procedure was not available in the hospital site of our research, and may have the disadvantage of making the grieving process more difficult (Magyari *et al.*, 1987).

Analysis of the transcripts of hospital consultations (see the section on *'Pregnancy Termination'* in Chapter 7) showed that doctors did not fully explain their pregnancy termination procedure, just as they did not discuss the nature of Down's syndrome, as shown in Chapter 1. For example, one doctor talked to two women about *'switching off'* a pregnancy. Those who stepped onto the risk escalator, for example by accepting serum screening, could not make fully informed decisions if they did not understand where it might take them.

Waiting for test results

Prenatal genetic screening/testing at our hospital research site entailed, at the time of the study, three possible waiting periods before the outcome was known: of one week for serum screening; of up to three weeks for amniocentesis; and of up to a month for the relatively high proportion of women who serum screen positive and then undergo amniocentesis (for example, 25 per cent of those aged over 37, as discussed in the Introduction). We have already noted, in the Introduction, the mixed evidence that screening positive causes pregnant women serious psychological distress. A pattern of high stress during the period of waiting for amniocentesis results followed by reassurance if they turn out negative has been found by Phipps and Zinn (1986); and by Evers-Kiebooms, Swerts and van den Berghe, (1988).

A 3 or 4-week wait for a definitive amniocentesis result might seem a small price to pay for the prevention of the birth of a baby with Down's syndrome. But this distressing waiting period may appear daunting to women contemplating it in the immediate future, and blot out longer-term concerns. The woman quoted below explained her refusal to accept serum screening in terms of the risk that, if she screened positive, she might then face a further wait for her amniocentesis result.

> **Pregnant woman:** *Well I thought, if I had the blood test, four out of five, there is one out of five high risk or something. And I thought, well, if I'm at high risk, then you are waiting. You go and have the amniocentesis, and you are waiting three weeks for that. And then they could say there is something wrong, but, at the end of the day, there might not be. So you've got all those months of chewing and preparing yourself, and then you have a normal baby. So why not have a nine month happy pregnancy, and then worry at the end of the day?* (Heather, aged 36, interview after taped hospital consultation [Bell], 18 weeks, no genetic tests)

Women who accepted genetic screening/testing did not always appreciate how much worry they might experience during the period of uncertainty. For those who had decided at the outset to abort a foetus with Down's syndrome, this waiting period could last for over half their pregnancy.

> **Previously pregnant midwife:** *It is an idea some of them come in and it is an idea – a friend up the road has had it done, and my friend has said it will put your mind at rest. But then, once they have the testing, they just don't seem to talk to other people. They keep that very secret which must be very hard as well, waiting for the results, especially with the amnios . . . It is a long time to wait.* (Jessica, midwife, aged 42, interview, post-partum, amniocentesis)

The following quotation suggests that even midwives may not fully appreciate the stress experienced by women waiting for test results.

> **Previously pregnant midwife:** *Well, it's hard because my friend who is a midwife had an amnio with her second one. She was 34 or 35 with [second child], and she came back, her serum screening came back 1 in 70. She plugged for amnio, and, of course, I was helping her, and supporting her, but watching her being so anxious until the phone call came*

through, everything was alright. And then, with her third one again, she was 38 by then, she decided rather than have serum screenings and be given a risk, she would just go for an amnio. (Tina, midwife, aged 37, interview, post-partum, serum screening)

This midwife had learnt about the anxiety which women may suffer whilst waiting for a high risk serum screening result to be followed up through her personal involvement, outside work, with a colleague. We may infer that she had not been directly exposed to this adverse experience in her professional role. Although she still decided to opt for serum screening, the above respondent could at least take this possibility into account when weighing up her options. Other women, like the next respondent quoted, did not anticipate how anxious they would feel.

Pregnant woman: *I would say I didn't enjoy it until I got the results of, you know the amnio, 'cos I had that done. Up until then it was just all worry, and I wouldn't like to go through that again now. The worry of the tests, the worry of a miscarriage, and then waiting four weeks for the results, that was awful. Didn't like that . . . And after the first ante-natal visit I just walked out, and I thought, 'I wish I hadn't got pregnant'. It was that bad, you know?* (Beatrice, aged 40, interview, 26 weeks, amniocentesis)

The respondent quoted below worried that her anxiety during the waiting period for amniocentesis results might adversely affect the health of her baby.

Interviewer: *How did you feel in the weeks that you were waiting for the results?*
Pregnant woman: *Oh it was awful. The result, waiting. It was just, it was, em, I was just crying and everything again, like I did when I found out I was pregnant. 'Cos I was saying, 'Ee, this baby will come out miserable little' . . . I mean, when you read the books and that, you think, 'Oh well, you know, three, four weeks'. But, like, you're wishing your life away, and it's awful, you know.* (Hilary, aged 40, interview, 23 weeks, amniocentesis)

Contemplating a risk can change it, a process we have described as reflexive recursion (Heyman and Henriksen, 1998b, pp. 94–103). This process can occur because thinking about a risk causes individuals to behave differently (Adams, 1995), or, in the case of health, because it is directly affected by emotional state. Women's heightened risk consciousness, stimulated by medical preventative procedures, may increase the risk of problems occurring in pregnancy (Mansfield, 1988). In addition, the above respondent's worry about such feedback effects itself contributed to the vortex of distress. The quotation also illustrates the way in which immediate considerations connected to longer-term concerns.

Because of the intensity of her anxiety, the woman quoted above held back from identifying with the baby, as found in other studies (Rothman, 1988; Heidrich and Cranley, 1989).

> **Interviewer:** *How did you feel towards the baby, whilst you were waiting for the results?*
> **Pregnant woman:** *Up until having the amnio, I never really thought I was pregnant, to tell you the truth. I was a bit like, 'Ah, I don't think it's me.' Even when I went to the hospital, you know, like to book in and that, I felt as though I was going for somebody else. And then, when I had the amnio done, and I could see the baby on the scan, then it brought it home to us, like. And then, after that, when I was waiting for the result, I was really frightened in case anything was the matter with it, you know, like really anxious.*(Hilary, aged 40, interview, 23 weeks, amniocentesis)

Her initial coping strategy of mildly dissociating herself from the woman who was pregnant was, ironically, disrupted by seeing the baby on the scan, an experience which triggered intense anxiety. Rothman (1994, p. 261) describes a new condition, *'a pregnancy without a baby'* which results from the suspension of maternal identification with the foetus until its genetic status has been assessed. As Lippman (1994, p. 22) notes, prenatal screening/testing *'separates a single entity, a pregnant woman, into two: herself, and her foetus'.* The barrier between self and foetus was shattered by the sight of the scan. White-van Mourik (1994) points out that modern diagnostic techniques have made foetal life both audible, through heart monitors, and visible, through ultrasound scans, to mothers much earlier than in the past, when the first sign of life would have been felt when the baby started kicking. She argues that these technical innovations have led to earlier bonding between mother and child, and so intensified maternal grief if the baby is lost. The genetic screening/testing system can, by creating uncertainty about the pregnancy outcome, work against the push towards earlier identification with the baby which arises as an unintended side-effect of scanning (Blumberg, 1984). Considerable internal tension may be experienced by women who have to manage these two opposed tendencies, as can be seen in the last quotation.

In contrast, women who rejected genetic screening/testing could identify with their baby from the time when they learnt about its conception.

> **Interviewer:** *Do you feel that the baby has been there, and yours throughout?*
> **Pregnant woman:** *I always classed* [it] *as a baby. I think, at the moment, it would still be classed as a foetus wouldn't it?*
> **Interviewer:** *Yes, that's really hard, when it's your baby.*
> **Pregnant woman:** *But I mean even when I found out, I mean, I was only 8 weeks, to me it was still a baby.* (Diane, aged 38, interview, 16 weeks, no genetic tests)

The choice of apparently similar words, usually without conscious reflection in everyday speech, can both convey and reinforce significant differences in attitude to the entity referenced. As Rothman (1988, p. 95) notes, attitudes are expressed *'in the tangled language of* **foetus** *and* **baby**' (quoted author's emphasis).

Miscarriage risk from amniocentesis

From a reproductive point of view, a miscarried foetus can usually be replaced. However, the consequent emotional distress may not be so easily recovered from. The following instructive quotation from a pregnant midwife illustrates the gap between these two perspectives. Her own experience of a miscarriage had enabled her to better appreciate the traumatic potential of this event.

> **Pregnant midwife:** *You don't, I mean, personally, I didn't think I would react so badly to having a miscarriage. And I've always thought of myself as being strong and dependable. I'm the one who keeps my husband propped up. And I just fell to pieces, and it is hard.* (Shirley, midwife, aged 34, interview, 20 weeks, no genetic tests)

Distress can last for a long time, and the above response illustrates the way in which medically short-term events might affect the future well beyond the pregnancy itself. Although she decisively rejected genetic screening/testing for herself, this midwife wished to keep this

rejection confidential, perhaps because she felt intuitively that it subverted one of the assumptions underlying the genetic risk prevention
system.

> **Pregnant midwife:** *Well, I miscarried in March, you see, so there was
> no way I was going to put this baby at risk* [by accepting amnio-
> centesis], *and you are talking about putting the baby at risk, really. But I
> wouldn't let anyone else know this, in my opinion.* (Shirley, midwife,
> aged 34, interview, 20 weeks, no genetic tests)

Gambling for peace of mind

Whatever they decided about genetic screening/testing, women had to
manage the uncertainty generated by selective attention to certain forms
of genetic risk. Those who opted for screening or testing had to pay the
price of heightened anxiety during the period of waiting for test results
in order, in most cases, to obtain a reduced probability of an adverse
outcome. They could, therefore, accept genetic tests in order to obtain
this early reassurance, rather than because they wanted to prevent the
birth of a child with Down's syndrome. The woman quoted below had
ruled out termination because she *'couldn't cope with terminating a
pregnancy after 20 weeks'* and rejected amniocentesis because of the risk
to the baby, but still opted for serum screening.

> **Pregnant woman:** *And if I had the serum screening test, that would
> let me know when it was high risk or a low risk. And if it were a low risk,
> well, I could practically rule out having a Down's baby anyway. So that
> was brilliant anyway, because that gave me peace of mind.* (Patricia, aged
> 37, interview, 24 weeks, serum screening)

This respondent, in effect, bought her immediate *'peace of mind'*
by gambling that she would receive a negative result which would
reduce her risk to a very low level. Since the majority of tests generate
negative results, this gamble will usually pay off. However, the probability of receiving a high risk serum screening result, about 15 per cent
for a woman aged 37 in the Northern Region (Northern Genetics
Service, 1998), is considerably higher than that of having a Down's
syndrome baby, about 1:240 for women of this age. If she had received
a positive result, having ruled out amniocentesis, this respondent
would have been faced with waiting for the birth in a state of
heightened anxiety.

The woman cited below, who had chosen amniocentesis, was more concerned about relieving the agony of present uncertainty than with preventing the birth of a baby with Down's syndrome.

Interviewer: *Why did you want the amnio?*

Pregnant woman: *The reason I wanted it is, because I don't think I could have gone until the baby's birth and not knowing if there's anything wrong with the baby.* (Beatrice, aged 40, interview, 26 weeks, amniocentesis)

Her strong need to bring forward the time when she would know the genetic status of her child persuaded this respondent to opt for amniocentesis, even though she *'hadn't made a definite decision'* about how she would respond to a positive result. The last two cases quoted demonstrate that shorter-term considerations could incline women to accept as well as, more commonly, to reject genetic screening and testing.

Longer-term considerations

Women who had definitely decided to accept pregnancy termination, if necessary, tended to adopt a long time-frame, justifying their decision in terms of the future prospects for the child and family, rather than focusing on the pregnancy itself. As discussed in Chapter 2, some older women felt that an age-related decline in vitality reduced their ability to cope with the care of a child with Down's syndrome. Hence, they associated maternal age with an increase in both the probability and the adversity of this contingency. However, women based their decisions on appraisal of the difficulties which they anticipated, and could not know how well they would actually cope with caring for a child with Down's syndrome. Van Riper, Ryff and Pridham (1992) found no evidence that caring for such a child affects family or parental well-being, or that either related to parental age. They advocate a competence model which proposes that parents learn to cope with the demands of caring for a child with a disability. But pregnant women may not take into account their own and their family's learning potential when they deliberate about genetic screening/testing.

Some respondents adopted time-frames which went well beyond the childhood of a baby with Down's syndrome. The woman quoted below balanced concern about her ability to cope when older against her fear of an amniocentesis-induced miscarriage.

Pregnant woman: *The thing is, in 20 years' time* [husband] *is going to be 67, and I'll be 60, you know. And we just don't know, we know we couldn't cope with it, you know. That's why I keep changing my mind about it, and keep thinking, 'Well, let's just get the amnio, and get it over with', you know. But then I know I would be heartbroken if we did.* (Marietta, aged 39, interview after taped hospital consultation [Laughton], 12 weeks, amniocentesis)

Some respondents adopted an even longer time-frame, weighing up the impact of giving birth to a baby with Down's syndrome on the adult lives of its siblings.

Interviewer: *Do you think you would have* [terminated pregnancy if amniocentesis result positive]?
Previously pregnant midwife: *I think I would have, yes. Especially with* [previous child] *because, then, you are thinking, my way of thinking is, an older parent, children outlive parents hopefully, but this one would be left to be cared for by his sibling. And it's the onus on the sibling I was thinking of more than us.* (Tina, midwife, aged 37, interview, postpartum, serum screening)

Appraisal of such long-term consequences could involve quite delicate calculations.

Interviewer: *Had you thought about what you would do if there had been a problem with the amnio?*
Pregnant woman: *I would have got rid of the baby, because, em, that one was very, very clear in my head, and it was clear with* [husband] *even though he was saying, 'Oh it will be alright', you know . . . I felt that I've got three kids . . . It shouldn't be their responsibility to look after their younger brother or sister if they were Down's syndrome or whatever . . . But I think I've got my kids into such a way. They are very compassionate, they are caring kids. You know that they would feel the way I would feel, that, if anything would happen to mum and dad, I would look after. And I wouldn't want that for them, to have that responsibility.* (Lesley, aged 37, interview, 26 weeks, amniocentesis)

This respondent's calculations took into account the likelihood that her children, because of their caring nature, would take responsibility in later life for a sibling with Down's syndrome. Rapp (1994), who explored the perspectives of American women about amniocentesis from an anthropological perspective, cited a similar example. An Italian-American Catholic homemaker had decided to abort after prenatal diagnosis of Down's syndrome on the grounds that she did not want her daughter's future life to be taken over by the obligation to look after her brother.

Predicting future intentions

The decision to accept genetic tests, even amniocentesis, did not entail a commitment to termination in the event that an abnormality was found, as we have seen. However, women who were motivated to take genetic tests primarily in order to prevent the birth of a child with genetic abnormalities were faced with the problem of predicting their own future intentions. For them, the main aim of screening/testing would be frustrated unless they were willing to accept an abortion if abnormalities were found. But they could not predict with certainty how they would react if this hypothetical, mostly unlikely, eventuality came to pass. In the same way, a healthy person cannot know for certain whether they would accept euthanasia if faced with a painful, terminal illness. Some women felt confident that they did not want a baby with genetic abnormalities, and would accept termination if necessary. Others doubted their own future intentions. Such uncertainty undermined the rationality of their acceptance of genetic screening/testing. The woman quoted below, a Catholic who had religious objections to abortion, coped with this problem by taking a step-by-step approach to decision-making which involved adopting a very short time-frame.

> **Previously pregnant midwife:** *And when we* [respondent and husband] *talked about it, you know, the what ifs, he said, 'Well, let's wait until we get the results.' And it would have been my decision what happened if we had a baby with Down's Syndrome. I don't know what decision I would have made.* (Jessica, aged 42, interview, post-partum, amniocentesis)

The next respondent, in contrast, attempted to predict the choice she would make if faced with a positive amniocentesis result, veering between rejection and acceptance of a hypothetical late termination.

> **Interviewer:** *Had you thought what you would do if there'd been a problem with the tests?* . . .

Pregnant woman: *I hadn't made a definite decision . . . But, by the time I went, the day I went for the results, I then thought, if there is something wrong, I don't know if I could do that. I think I still would have terminated, to be honest. But, I mean, it would have been, it wouldn't have been very nice. There's no easy way out, it's really hard, you know.* (Beatrice, aged 40, interview, 26 weeks, amniocentesis)

Exposure to the doubts of others could intensify uncertainty about one's own intentions.

Interviewer: *Had you thought further of what you would have done. Had you thought about the results of the amnio?*
Pregnant woman: *Aha. It's awful, 'cos you think, like, it's fair enough having the decision of the amnio. And then, like, me husband was saying, 'Well what happens after that?', if the decision was not the right decision, you know. I don't think I could have went ahead with the pregnancy, to be honest.* (Hilary, aged 40, interview, 23 weeks, amniocentesis)

Even women who had made their minds up to definitely terminate if an abnormality was discovered could find themselves uncertain about their own intentions later in the pregnancy process.

Pregnant woman: *And that was when I was talking to people and saying, ee, I know I was so positive at the beginning, if there's something wrong, em, I'm going to get rid of it. But when it came to the actual crunch, in that three weeks, the baby was moving lots, em, the sickness had stopped to the point of I wasn't feeling nausea. So everything was settling, em, and it was like, ee, could I really get rid of it now? So that was very worrying.* (Lesley, aged 37, interview, 26 weeks, amniocentesis)

A woman who accepted the perceived risk of an amniocentesis-induced miscarriage in order to prevent the birth of a child with Down's syndrome would take this risk for no purpose if she was not prepared to go through with a termination. But women could not know how they would feel later in their pregnancy at the time when they accepted amniocentesis. The next respondent had realised that uncertainty about how she would respond if a risk turned into a reality undermined the utilitarian calculation on which her decision to accept serum screening had been based.

> **Pregnant woman:** *I suppose I was naive* [in previous pregnancy] *in the fact that I didn't know how I would have reacted if they had said, 'Well, you are high risk.' But somehow in the back of your mind, you had the confidence they were not going to say that. Just because it was a simple enough test. It did not carry a risk of anything else.* (Linda, aged 39, interview after hospital consultation [Loftus], 14 weeks, amniocentesis)

Her suspension of forward planning was predicated on the assumption that an adverse contingency with a relatively low probability, assessed through an apparently simple test, would not occur. She discounted this probability as effectively zero, and so could treat serum screening as costless.

Uncertainty about one's own future feelings could also undermine the rationality of the irreversible decision to undergo an abortion.

> **Pregnant woman:** *I don't think people appreciate, or the profession appreciates, the aftermath of a termination anyway, whether that baby has been wanted but is disabled and they can't face it, or they think they don't want it and terminate . . . I have a couple of friends who have had terminations, and they are shattered. It has totally changed their lives. No matter how much they couldn't have that baby, they wished to God that they had it, do you know what I mean, having it and living with it.* (Elizabeth, aged 25, interview after taped hospital consultation [Fallowfield], 13 weeks, no genetic tests)

Such reactions extended the adversity of a termination into the longer term, as already noted with respect to miscarriages.

Some women felt confident about their own intentions, for example having decided to definitely abort a foetus with Down's syndrome.

> **Pregnant woman:** *We obviously want to know* [the results] *as soon as possible, so we don't want to get anything* [for the baby] *if the baby has got to be terminated* (Mary, aged 46, interview after taped hospital consultation [Anderson], 16 weeks, amniocentesis)

The rationality of such decision-making depended upon the extent to which women could correctly predict their intentions in various hypothetical futures. The last woman quoted, whose experiences will be further discussed at the end of the chapter, unfortunately, had to decide whether to go through with termination when Down's syndrome was detected. She did so, but with considerable anguish and uncertainty.

Pregnant woman: *And* [the doctor] *says that we could go home and think about it, or come back. Well we had already made up* [our minds]. *If I'd gone home . . . I wouldn't have come back to hospital the next day.* (Mary, aged 46, interview after pregnancy termination, 17 weeks, amniocentesis)

The finding that women are more likely to opt for termination after a positive amniocentesis result if it is given by a geneticist than if it is communicated by an obstetrician (Holmes-Seidle, Ryynanen and Lindembaum, 1987) testifies to the tentative status of decisions made in adverse, not previously experienced circumstances.

Doctors' attitudes towards temporal commitment varied considerably. Some women felt pressurised to agree in advance to a termination if Down's syndrome was detected.

Previously pregnant midwife: *I said to the consultant that I would like one* [amniocentesis test], *but I didn't know what action I would take if the baby was abnormal. So* [the doctor] *said think about it, and . . . talk to* [the doctor] *again the next time. So I don't think* [the doctor] *was prepared to do it without me saying I would have an abortion . . . I told* [the doctor] *I wanted to get my way.* (Jessica, midwife, aged 42, interview, post-partum, amniocentesis)

Her status as a midwife may have given this woman the confidence to resist making a promise which she might not have been able to keep. The doctor cited below offered a different perspective on decision timing from that illustrated in the last quotation.

Doctor: *We used to say that there is no point having the test* [amniocentesis] *if you would not want to terminate the pregnancy if there was a problem. But we have gone away from that, because some people feel they would like to know so that they would be able to cope better at the end* (Mary, aged 46, hospital consultation [Anderson], 15 weeks, amniocentesis)

On this view, women who had ruled out termination might opt for screening or testing simply for informational purposes, to bring forward the time of knowing the genetic status of their baby, and so facilitate coping.

Women who chose initial serum screening also needed to assess what they might do if they screened negative or positive. Doctors, again, expressed conflicting opinions about whether a woman who had received a negative, low risk serum screening result could subsequently be given amniocentesis. The quotation below ruled out this possibility.

> **Doctor:** *If you start off definitely wanting to know whether this baby definitely has got Down's syndrome, then, and you are not going to be pacified with a chance result, then there is no point in having a blood test done. You should have amniocentesis.* (Penny, aged 36, hospital consultation [Lewin], 12 weeks, amniocentesis)

Choice of the term *'pacified'* may have conveyed to the woman that the doctor viewed the need for certainty as unreasonable, and this attitude may have contributed towards her indecision. At the end of the hospital consultation, this woman said that she needed *'a bit more time'* to decide but that she thought she would *'have the blood test'*. However, she eventually selected amniocentesis at a relatively young age for this hospital, perhaps, in part, because the doctor's choice of words made her doubt whether a low risk serum screening result would give her peace of mind. In contrast, the opening up by the doctor of the option of amniocentesis after a negative serum screening result may have helped the next woman quoted to begin the preventative process with serum screening rather than amniocentesis.

> **Doctor:** *Even if you had a normal test result, we are not saying, just because you had a normal blood test, you can't have the amnio. It's a screen test, and it gives you an idea of where you want to go next.* (Maria, aged 36, hospital consultation [Bell], 11 weeks, serum screening)

If this option, which licensed a step-by-step approach to decision timing, was ruled out, women were, in effect, asked to predict how they would feel about their level of risk serum test result. Our qualitative data shows that some women felt uncertain about their ability to do so. The finding of one Finnish study (Santalahti *et al.*, 1999), mentioned previously, that the proportion of women who said they would decline to terminate a pregnancy if a disorder such as Down's syndrome was discovered was nearly double the proportion who actually declined (13 per cent), suggests that this uncertainty is well founded.

Screening/testing outcomes

The right-hand part of Figure 3.1 displays alternative possible genetic screening/testing outcomes. Our survey did not include questions on test results, and, in any event, reliable results could not have been obtained from a survey of 1500 pregnancies, given the low underlying Down's syndrome prevalence in the population. However, we have been able to combine the survey results about women's choices with statistical estimates of average, maternal age-related rates of Down's syndrome.

Figure 3.1 shows that the hospital was reasonably successful at filtering out cases of Down's syndrome whilst screening/testing only a minority of pregnant women. Only 10 per cent (161) of the sample were offered, and 7 per cent (108) underwent, some form of genetic test. Given their age distribution, just one live birth per 6000 pregnancies would be expected among women who did not proceed as far as obtaining a definitive diagnosis through amniocentesis. One to two babies with Down's syndrome would be expected among the 33 women who received amniocentesis either initially or as a result of a positive serum screening result.

Serum screening outcomes

The detective success outlined above was obtained at some cost. We have estimated that about 12 women would have been classified as at higher risk after serum screening, and that 10 of these women would have proceeded to amniocentesis. Most of those who screened positive could have avoided both the distress of being located in a higher risk group and the possible risk of miscarriage from amniocentesis, whilst still giving birth to a baby with normal chromosomes.

Finally, we may note two byways in the decision maze represented in Figure 3.1. As illustrated above, some doctors emphasised, in the hospital consultation, that women who opted for serum screening could still choose amniocentesis even if the result of the former test showed that they were at low risk. Our model suggests that, in practice, women were very unlikely to take up this option, an assessment with which the hospital doctors concurred. We have also assumed, on the basis of other estimates, that about 20 per cent of women whom serum screening places in the higher risk group will not proceed to amniocentesis (Dawson *et al.*, 1993; Northern Genetics Service, 1998).

Amniocentesis

We have already illustrated the relief felt by women who received negative amniocentesis results. Our sample included one case of a woman, aged 46, who, unfortunately, received a positive amniocentesis result, and decided upon a termination. She and her husband agreed to be interviewed four months after the termination. Despite sensitive care by hospital staff, this couple had found the whole experience traumatic. They expected the damage caused to their well-being to extend well into the future.

The father described the doctor who broke the news as *'really great'* whilst the mother described this doctor as *'lovely'*. The couple were not pressured into going ahead with the termination, although the mother felt uncertain about her own resolve in such extreme circumstances, as noted above. They had made it clear at the hospital consultation, which was transcribed, that they had already decided to terminate the pregnancy if anything was *'seriously wrong'*. The preventative system had 'worked' by both meeting the parents' wishes and avoiding the birth of a child with Down's syndrome. Nevertheless, they paid a high price for this medical success.

The mother described feeling *'so empty'* and *'lost'*, and both parents experienced a weakened sense of reality.

> **Father:** *To me it was like a dream, as though, you know, feel all hazy all over things like that, hazy around my head.*
> **Mother:** *But I was, keep nipping myself, thinking.*
> **Father:** *In a daze.* (Mary, aged 46, interview after pregnancy termination, 17 weeks, amniocentesis)

Cohen (1993) describes the temporal fissure which opens up in their lives when parents discover that their child has a serious illness, an experience which one parent described as *'walking through the gates of hell'* (p. 83). As well as grieving, our parents had to live with intense feelings of guilt and anger. Even though the genetic screening system aims to detect and destroy (to put it bluntly) genetically abnormal foetuses, the mother still feared that she might be vilified by hospital staff.

> **Mother:** *I was frightened of being judged by the hospital, you know. I was frightened that the nurses would judge me, and think that I was killing my baby, you know, which I was doing, but it was for the best.* (Mary, aged 46, interview after pregnancy termination, 17 weeks, amniocentesis)

This guilt was intensified, at the time of the abortion, by panicky fear that the diagnosis of genetic abnormality might have been mistaken.

> **Mother:** *I wake up from a terrible bad dream – they're only kidding us about my baby . . . And on the Sunday, when I had him, I was terrified in case they had made a mistake, and he was alright when he came out . . . But he wasn't. You could see he was Down's . . .* (Mary, aged 46, interview after pregnancy termination, 17 weeks, amniocentesis)

This nightmare was predicated on awareness of the fallibility, notwithstanding its claims to the contrary, of modern science.

The couple helped themselves to come to terms with their decision by affirming the poverty of the life prospects for a child with Down's syndrome. They reacted against a representation of the birth of a baby with Down's syndrome as a positive event.

> **Mother:** *I read a story. Reading this story has helped me cope with it . . . I think they are bloody stupid. It's in 'Take a Break' . . . They look like they are really over the moon because they are having this Down's baby.*
> **Father:** *I mean they will have been explained the same as everybody else as to what can happen, or what it is going to be like, and what it means for the future.*
> **Mother:** *They can have chest infections.*
> **Father:** *There's any number of things that we know that can happen . . .*
> **Mother:** *I mean they are laughed and they are scorned at.* (Mary, aged 46, interview after pregnancy termination, 17 weeks, amniocentesis)

As well as trying to deal with a sense of guilt, both parents had to manage intense anger that such an adverse event had happened to them, and not to somebody else.

> **Mother:** *I wish, I wanted him so much, and what made matters worse was, the girl next door, her daughter was expecting, is expecting a baby at the same time as mine. I hated* [neighbour] *on that day on the Sunday, Saturday, I hated her . . . Why should I be the 30th one, you know? Why couldn't it have been somebody else?* (Mary, aged 46, interview after pregnancy termination, 17 weeks, amniocentesis)

This question exposes a central limitation of the inductive probability heuristic (Heyman, Henriksen and Maughan, 1998), discussed in Chapter 4, that it cannot predict which individuals within a category will experience an event of which the aggregate rate has been estimated.

Feelings of loss, guilt and anger inevitably create barriers which make everyday relationships difficult. The mere pervasiveness of babies in the environment may cause intense pain.

> **Mother:** *And I think, everywhere I go, there's loads of babies.* (Mary, aged 46, interview after pregnancy termination, 17 weeks, amniocentesis)

The parents both felt permanently damaged by their experience. At the time of the interview, at least, they saw the termination as having long-term consequences.

> **Father:** *I feel I've aged ten years. I feel shattered. I mean, I am shattered. I've hardly slept, and things like that, chewing over the facts of why of, sort of why, how, you know, could it happen again? And if it does, you know, I mean we've got to go through it again.* (Husband of Mary, aged 46, interview after pregnancy termination, 17 weeks, amniocentesis)

We cannot necessarily generalise from one case. Every couple who agree to terminate a pregnancy will respond differently. However, a similar picture of loss, grief, uncertainty about the decision to terminate and disruption of everyday relationships has been painted in a number of studies of women's responses to terminating a pregnancy on account of genetic abnormalities (Donnai, Charles and Harris, 1981; Furlong and Black, 1984; Jones *et al.*, 1984; White-van Mourik *et al.*, 1992). Such findings bring into question the brutal but revealing assumption made by one group of health economists that termination costs parents nothing because *'the replacement rate of a lost foetus, following an induced or spontaneous abortion, is 100 percent'* (Beazoglou *et al.*, 1998, p. 1242).

We may anticipate that the grief, guilt and anger experienced by this couple might abate over time. And we may suggest that those who are involved in an intense emotional experience find it difficult to empathise with a future self who will have travelled some temporal distance from the disturbing event. Black (1989) found that the proportion of women who felt able to resume normal work and social activities increased from about 70 per cent one month after the termination to 80 per cent after six months. A small but statistically significant decline in perceived partner support over this period was observed. Over a longer time-span, White-van Mourik (1992) concluded that, two years after the event, most parents felt at peace with themselves about their decision to terminate a pregnancy because abnormalities had been discovered. But 20 per cent of women still reported feelings such as anger, guilt and distress. Laurence (1989) found that about 80 per cent of women who underwent a termination for genetic reasons experienced an acute grief reaction, and that nearly half were still grieving six months later. Only 1 in 20 reacted in this way following spontaneous abortion or termination for medical-social reasons.

These findings suggest that women who undergo voluntary, late termination face a substantial risk of suffering emotional harm. However, this risk, a remote possibility at the point in time at which they were considering genetic screening/testing for most women, was not discussed with them during the hospital consultation. It lurked at the end of a risk escalator which might begin with an apparently innocent blood test.

6
The Hospital Consultation I: The Pre-test Risk of Genetic Abnormalities

Introduction

The next two chapters will explore issues arising from the hospital consultation, drawing on qualitative analysis of transcripts of 16 hospital consultations, carried out by six consultants and three registrars working at the hospital site for our research. This analysis will be supported, where possible, by quotations from post-consultation interviews undertaken with ten of these pregnant women. (The other six did not consent to a follow-up interview, or could not be contacted.) The combination of direct observation of consultation content with access to women's interpretations of what they had been told through the post-consultation interviews provided a powerful methodology for understanding the communication of genetic information in the hospital consultation.

The sample of hospital consultations

Women who met specific selection criteria in terms of their age and the doctor referred to were approached by their midwife and asked to give informed consent for their hospital consultation to be transcribed, which none declined. Thirteen of the 16 participants, including the respondent, discussed at the end of Chapter 5, who terminated her pregnancy after a positive amniocentesis result, were aged 35 and over (range 35–46 years). Three younger women, aged 25–27, one of whom eventually opted for serum screening, were included in this sample so that contrasts could be drawn between the interactions of doctors with women above and below the operational higher risk age boundary of 35. Four of the 16 women, aged 25–39, received no genetic tests; five, aged 27–38, underwent serum screening; and seven women, aged 36–46, underwent amniocentesis.

Apart from in the cases summarised below, women's eventual choice of test matched the intention stated in the hospital interview. One woman, aged 36, stated at interview that she would probably opt for serum screening, but ended up taking amniocentesis. The other, aged 39, indicated at the consultation that she had decided on amniocentesis, but was not tested. Three women, one aged 27 who was serum screened, and two aged 36 and 39 who received amniocentesis, did not express a clear intention at the consultation.

The consultations

The discussions lasted, on average, for about seven minutes, with a mean total of 1440 words spoken (range 590–2709). Doctors generated 90 per cent of the words spoken. The above statistics reveal the character of these transactions, as mostly brief information-giving sessions driven by the doctor's agenda. Consultants would have preferred to offer women fuller discussion provided by trained genetic counsellors, but were unable to fund this service, as noted in the Introduction. During informal discussions, doctors stated that their own efforts were constrained by heavy workloads and lack of training in counselling. As also noted in the Introduction, we refer to their talks with women about prenatal genetic screening/testing as 'consultations' and not as 'counselling sessions'.

Health professionals who advise pregnant women and their partners are faced with a demanding informational task which they may struggle to accomplish. Burn *et al.* (1996) found that 40 per cent of pregnant women who had received prenatal serum screening in one maternity unit would have liked more information; and that this proportion was reduced, but not eliminated, by measures designed to improve communication, use of a video and provision of a co-ordinator to train midwives.

Scope of Chapters 6 and 7

The analysis presented in the next two chapters will explore the following issues: the opening gambits through which doctors set the agenda for the hospital consultation; the representation of pre-test genetic risks; the genetic screening/testing decision tree and its navigation; and, finally, the impact of serum screening and amniocentesis on the risk picture.

As in the pioneering study of Lippman-Hand and Fraser (1979a, b), which encompassed a range of genetic conditions, we will compare, wherever possible, hospital consultation transcripts with women's retrospective accounts of their meaning. This powerful combination brings social scientists, in collaboration with their research participants, just about as close as they can get to observing the interpretation of ecologically meaningful interactions. However, unlike Lippman-Hand and Fraser, we will focus not so much on the heuristics through which pregnant women comprehended complex risk pictures, but on the simplifications which doctor and pregnant woman managed jointly. The interpretive labour of doctors who provided genetic advice at our hospital will be analysed at least as closely as that of pregnant women. We will show, for example, that doctors often, but not always, treated Down's syndrome as a homogenous, well-defined condition (see also Chapter 1); and simplified the four types of probability outlined in Table 0.2 (of Down's syndrome given a screen positive or negative, and of a screen positive or negative given Down's syndrome).

Opening gambits

The way in which a doctor opened the discussion set the agenda, defining the problem(s) of concern. We will explore variations in the opening move, and speculate about their possible influence on a woman's eventual choice of screening/testing option.

The opening gambit for younger women

Women aged under 35 were, at our hospital research site, classified as being at low risk of giving birth to a baby with Down's syndrome, unless a personal or family history of chromosomal problems had been identified. They were not usually offered a discussion of genetic screening/testing (see Chapter 3). Doctors started each of the three transcribed sessions with younger women by minimising their Down's syndrome risk, steering them away from genetic screening/testing. One woman aged 25 was concerned about a family history of spina bifida and hydrocephalus. The doctor who conducted this consultation informed the woman that the above problems would be picked up reliably in the scan, and that, therefore, serum screening was not indicated. The consultation opened as follows:

> **Doctor:** *Do you have any problems?*
> **Pregnant woman:** *Just with my mother's history, of my brother having spina bifida and hydrocephaly. He never lived but I was offered the Alpha Feto-Protein test.* (Elizabeth, aged 25, hospital consultation [Fallowfield], 12 weeks, no genetic tests)

The doctor went on to dismiss serum screening as not *'appropriate'*, and to tell her that *'as far as we know, neural defects are not familial'*. This woman might not have found the scientific caution contained in the phrase *'as far as we know'* reassuring. Nevertheless, we may link the moderately woman-centred opening gambit, not found in any of the other interviews, to this doctor's strategic aim of diverting this woman from a path which the doctor considered inappropriate. By passing agenda-setting to her, the doctor encouraged her to express her own beliefs, and lay them open to expert correction.

The doctor opened another consultation with a younger woman by excluding her from the higher risk group, as *'a little bit of particularly low risk from the spina bifida and also Down's'* (Lucy, aged 27 [Loftus], hospital consultation, 12 weeks, no genetic tests). In the third recorded session, with a woman also aged 27, the doctor began the consultation by focusing on screening procedures, asking her *'How much do you know about the test?'* (Ruth, aged 27 [Laughton], hospital consultation, 12 weeks, serum screening). This approach was often used with older women, and took the desirability of screening/testing for granted. We cannot demonstrate that this woman accepted serum screening at an unusually young age because the doctor took this approach. As noted in Chapter 3, doctors may have, in some cases matched their opening gambits to women's prior intentions. For example, they were more likely to offer genetic tests to worried women. About 80 per cent of women reported, in a retrospective survey, that they had made their decision about genetic screening/testing before the first hospital consultation (Sullivan and Kirk, 1999). Whatever the direction of influence, congruence between the three above decisions and the doctor's approach to the consultation can be identified.

The opening gambit for older women

In contrast, doctors advising older women usually set the agenda around genetic risks. For example, the opening move given below used a pre-consultation question about scans to introduce the doctor's concern about the age-related risk of Down's syndrome.

> **Doctor:** *You asked what indications we might see from your scan.*
> **Pregnant woman:** *Yes. Obviously, at this stage, it's probably too early, but I'm aware that there are certain indicators that would show.*
> **Doctor:** *All I would like to say to you is that there are hard signs and soft signs . . . Now I wouldn't say to you that any of the signs that we've*

got from ultrasound are particularly, well, they aren't particularly indicative, to be honest with you, with Down's syndrome.
Pregnant woman: *Right.*
Doctor: *You are 36. Do you know what the risk is of you having a baby with Down's Syndrome?* (Charlotte, aged 36, hospital consultation [Fallowfield], 12 weeks, amniocentesis)

The doctor's response directed attention away from this woman's question about immediately available information from the scan, and towards the risk of Down's syndrome. The doctor went on to inform her in some technical detail, not included in the quotation, that scans provide only a limited indicator for this condition. The length of this presentation, and its follow-up with a question about her knowledge of the risk of Down's syndrome, must have conveyed to this woman that she faced a serious risk. Her response suggests that she had previously felt uncertain about the severity of this problem.

Doctor: *Is it* [Down's syndrome] *something that you are worried about?*
Pregnant woman: *No. It's just that, obviously, having just turned 36, I'm not neurotic by any means, but you do think, and you see where the levels are, where you, where the dangers increase. And friends of a similar age, slightly older, have had blood tests, have had amnio, and it just makes you think, 'Well, maybe it's something I should think about, and go away and decide'.*
Doctor: *Yes, OK . . .*
Pregnant woman: *I mean my own doctor said, 'Don't be so stupid, bugger off.'* (Charlotte, aged 36, hospital consultation [Fallowfield], 12 weeks, amniocentesis)

This woman's denial of neuroticism, and semi-humorous recitation of her GP's dismissal of her fears, convey her initial uncertainty. The opening gambit in the consultation may have tilted the balance towards fear of age-related risks, and towards acceptance of amniocentesis at a relatively young age. Choice of the term *'danger'*, rather than risk, reflects this concern. Risks may be appraised, whilst dangers should be avoided (Heyman and Huckle, 1993). Her anxiety led her to locate herself in a *'slightly older'* age group who had been tested.

As repeatedly emphasised, the influence of the doctor who gives genetic advice should not be exaggerated, or linked too closely to women's decisions with the misleading benefit of hindsight. Doctors may attempt to support a woman by slanting material towards her presumed stance. In the above example, we can see that the doctor's concern about Down's syndrome resonated with this woman's prior anxiety. Her own comments, in an interview carried out after the hospital consultation, confirm this impression.

Interviewer: *From the interview* [with hospital doctor], *I really didn't, I wasn't sure whether you had decided to have the amniocentesis.*

Pregnant woman: *I decided, I think, in my mind, I virtually decided that I would have it. I just wanted somebody to tell me that, yes, to have it done was the right thing to do you know.* (Charlotte, aged 36, interview after hospital consultation [Fallowfield], 16 weeks, amniocentesis)

The hospital doctor had not overtly advised this woman that amniocentesis was *'the right thing to do'*, as she suggested, and had emphasised that *'it's a personal decision'*. But she had understood the doctor to have recommended amniocentesis. Comparison with the following example, in which a woman of a similar age opted not to be tested, illustrates the way in which a very different initial tone to the consultation could be set.

Doctor: *You've got three children, right?*
Pregnant woman: *Yes.*
Doctor: *And how old are they? The oldest is 12?*
Pregnant woman: *17, 15 and 12.*
Doctor: *The youngest is 12, sorry. OK. And you had quite normal pregnancies? . . . What we need to do, with your permission, is to give you a scan just to check the dates. Not to look to make sure that there are problems, but to see the baby. There's no problem with that. And we can use that for the basis for our chat about age-related testing. How old are you, 36? Are you a smoker? Have you managed to reduce it at all? Have you been trying or not?*
Pregnant woman: *Yes.*
Doctor: *Up to date with your smears? Otherwise fit and well? Are you working?* (Heather, aged 36 [Bell], hospital consultation, 16 weeks, no genetic tests)

The opening move in this consultation set a framework of normality. The woman is reminded of the unproblematic nature of her previous pregnancies. The aim of the initial scan is defined as merely age-setting, with the detection of abnormalities specifically ruled out. Even the reference to smoking might provide reassurance, since it links the outcome of the pregnancy to lifestyle factors within the woman's control, rather than to unalterable, partly random genetic mutations. Quick-fire questioning put maternal age-related genetic risks in a wider context of other types of normality. (However, as noted in Chapter 1, the desirability of screening scans, which the doctor recommended as *'very good at picking up spina bifida and related conditions, serious problems'* was taken for granted.)

In an interview following the hospital consultation, this respondent stated that she *'knew what I would do'*, before the consultation. Although she felt that the doctor *'gave both sides really'*, the main message which she had retained concerned the risk of false positives, and so was in tune with the doctor's opening emphasis on normality.

Pregnant woman: [The doctor] *said that some people think it is better not to do it* [serum screening] *..., that it's more stress because there might not be anything wrong with it even if it comes up positive.* (Heather, aged 36, interview after taped hospital consultation [Bell], 18 weeks, no genetic tests)

The opening quoted below from another session, conducted by the same doctor with a woman of similar age, suggests that a doctor's opening gambit could vary considerably.

Doctor: *Alright, I'll just go and get the details for 36. Have a look at that, the age-related risk.*
Pregnant woman: *It's just with our* [previous child] *being alright, because I am getting a bit older, and it does worry me.* (Maria, aged 36, hospital consultation [Bell], 11 weeks, serum screening)

The doctor opened the previously quoted session by emphasising the normality of the pregnancy, but began the present consultation by homing in on age-related risks. The woman's response shows that she accepted this concern. As already noted, doctors may tailor their information-giving strategy to the anticipated views of the women they are advising, perhaps unconsciously, whilst uncertain women may respond to the tone which their medical adviser sets. However, since doctors are only human, we cannot rule out the influence of personal factors such as mood. Their approach to the complex matter of communicating about genetic risks and screening/testing options are likely to be affected by numerous influences, of which the science is only one.

In the above cases, the doctor's opening line appeared to have been either taken up by the pregnant woman or tailored to their pre-existing preferences. Occasionally, women rejected medical advice. The doctor quoted below suggested that, at most, the lesser procedure of serum screening was needed.

> **Doctor:** *Right, at the age of 36, you really are on the borderline of the age group at which we would offer screening, for Down's syndrome, which is what we are really talking about when you talk about this sort of screening.* (Penny, aged 36, hospital consultation [Lewin], 12 weeks, amniocentesis)

During the interview, the doctor appeared to favour initial serum screening, which the woman opted for at that time. However, she eventually underwent amniocentesis. Women did not passively accept implicit or explicit advice, although they may well have been influenced by the doctor's attitude if initially uncertain.

Although the opening gambit could vary, most hospital consultations for older women began from the same premise: that the woman faced a serious medical problem because of her age-related risk of Down's syndrome, and, therefore, needed to make a difficult choice between imperfect screening/testing options. The gravity with which their situation could be represented is illustrated in the following quotations.

> **Doctor:** *Get yourself ready, and we'll have a chat about age-related risks.* (Joan, aged 37, hospital consultation [Bell], 11 weeks, amniocentesis)
> **Doctor:** *I know you will have had all sorts of thoughts and even nightmares about what to do in terms of screening. What are your thoughts?* (Linda, aged 39 [Loftus], hospital consultation, 12 weeks, amniocentesis)
> **Doctor:** *You are just 36 years old?*
> **Pregnant woman:** *Yes, that's right. Yes, just gone.*
> **Doctor:** *We do discuss the problem with screening for a chromosome abnormality with anybody 36 and over. I have got to tell you, you are just 36. If you were just not 36, we would not be having this discussion.* (Sarah, aged 36, hospital consultation [Dickson], 10 weeks, amniocentesis)

The first doctor quoted advised the pregnant woman to brace herself for bad news, although this impression was softened through characterisation of the intended discussion as a *'chat'*. The second doctor associated screening with *'nightmares'*, whilst the third suggested that, at the age of 36, the woman has crossed a boundary into a danger zone. Again, the choice of language, in this case *'I have got to tell you'*, implied that bad news was about to be delivered, even though a merely conventional, boundary, variably defined even within a single hospital, between higher and lower risk categories had been crossed.

Doctors problematised maternal age as a risk factor for Down's syndrome. They rarely represented the pregnancy of an older woman as a positive event. Even when the pregnancy was celebrated, the doctor's positive tone could be qualified by a reference to the risk of Down's syndrome.

> **Doctor:** *I bet you were delighted right from the start . . . You are interested in knowing your risk of having a Down's Syndrome baby?*
> **Pregnant woman:** *Yes.* (Marietta, aged 39, hospital consultation [Laughton], 10 weeks, amniocentesis)

The woman's agenda

Because doctors focused so clearly, and so early, on genetic risks, older women were given little opportunity to raise their own concerns. Only two of the 16 women whose hospital consultations were transcribed asked questions about issues other than genetic screening/testing. One woman was provided with reassurance about the risks associated with maternal German measles. The second woman asked about her chance of having twins, but her doctor responded by relating this concern to the risk of Down's syndrome.

> **Doctor:** *Ask me any questions you think of, and make a decision about what you are doing, nothing, the amniocentesis or the blood test.*
> **Pregnant woman:** *Okay. The only thing, I'm not worried, but I would like to know about my baby, is the chance of it being twins. I'm a twin and my cousin had, the midwife did say that it might be a probability.*
> **Doctor:** *Yes. If there is twins that complicates, if there is a problem. Usually, there is a family history of twins, and it increases your risk of a twin having problems, say a 1 in 80 chance* [of Down's syndrome], *almost doubles your chance . . . Now all this takes the fun out of the pregnancy, doesn't it?*
> **Pregnant woman:** *It does a bit.* (Marietta, aged 39, hospital consultation [Laughton], 10 weeks, amniocentesis)

This instructive quotation illustrates the powerful influence of the genetic screening/testing agenda on the course of the consultation. A question about the probability of giving birth to twins was heard as asking about the risk of a twin having Down's syndrome. The doctor wryly noted that consideration of genetic risks *'takes the fun out of pregnancy'*, a sentiment with which the pregnant woman could only agree. A gap between genetic counsellor and counsellee perceptions of objectives was also detected by Michie and Marteau (1996) in a small pilot study, with counsellors most frequently assuming that clients sought information about occurrence probabilities and tests. Armstrong, Michie and Marteau (1998) found that genetic counsellors' interactional styles, involving standardisation of the agenda and use of closed questions, prevented clients from raising their own concerns.

The pre-test risk picture

As was argued in the Introduction, risk assessments are based on the synthesis of probabilistic beliefs with value judgements about future event classes which are treated as if they are homogenous, and selectively attended to, within a time-frame set by individuals. The value component in a risk assessment may be taken for granted, with the result that probability and risk are treated as equivalent. This backgrounding of value questions can be identified in the hospital consultations, since the meaning of Down's syndrome was discussed only briefly, if at all, whilst the probability of its occurrence, and how this probability could be managed, were discussed in some depth.

The meaning of Down's syndrome

Although doctors focused the hospital consultation agenda on the risk of Down's syndrome, they did not explore the nature and health implications of this highly variable condition, as noted in Chapter 1. Doctors and pregnant women discussed the probability of an event which was bracketed as highly negative. The discussions were predicated on a shared understanding which was simply, and perhaps unjustifiably, taken for granted.

Pregnant women's understanding of the intellectual and health problems associated with Down's syndrome was explored in only two of the 16 transcribed hospital consultations, whilst the probability of this condition was discussed in all of them. Other studies have also shown that the nature of the conditions being tested for tends not to be discussed in risk consultations. Marteau *et al.* (1992a) found that the conditions being tested for (Down's syndrome and neural tube defects) were discussed in only four out of 102 consultations with midwives and obstetricians, a finding which closely matches that of our smaller, qualitative study. Similarly, Rapp (1988) found, in a participant observation study, that trained genetic counsellors, who had internalised a medical perspective, did not discuss the meaning of Down's syndrome, its variability or sensitivity to environmental influences. Such findings suggest that the tendency to bracket and take for granted both the nature of and public knowledge about constituted risk entities such as Down's syndrome is deep-seated.

The two discussions of Down's syndrome which did take place in the consultations drew selective attention to the condition whilst, at the same time, raising the question of what it meant. However, the first of these openings offered no more than a token reference to the meaning of Down's syndrome, since the doctor did not provide any further information on this topic despite the pregnant woman's admission of ignorance.

> **Doctor:** *Have you read anything about DS* [Down's syndrome] *yet?*
> **Pregnant woman:** *No. Just what was in the booklet.*
> **Doctor:** *I think there are two ways we can look at what we are going to do about it. There is the blood test. What the BT* [blood test] *does, it tells you if you are at high risk or at low risk . . .* (Hazel, aged 38, hospital consultation [Crabtree], 8 weeks, serum screening)

This quotation illustrates how rapid removal of the phenomenon to be prevented from clinical discourse enables risk to be equated with probability in the practice of health care. The one hospital consultation in which the nature of Down's syndrome was raised as an issue stands out as anomalous.

> **Doctor:** *So the first thing is do you know what Down's syndrome is?*
> **Pregnant woman:** *No.*
> **Doctor:** *A condition where there are chromosomal abnormalities, where the babies, to a greater or lesser extent, have mental retardation which can't be predicted. And not all of them, but some of them, have abnormalities like heart defects. That's what it is, and I think you will have seen children affected by it.*
> **Pregnant woman:** *Yeah.*
> **Doctor:** *And who else has had a baby with Down's syndrome?*

Pregnant woman: *It is my husband's aunt.*
Doctor: *Your husband's aunt. Now, the first thing is, do you remember how old she was when she had the baby?*
Pregnant woman: *About 42.*
Doctor: *Down's is something that generally does not run in families.*
(Susan, aged 35, hospital consultation [Gould], 15 weeks, serum screening)

Even in this exceptional case, the brief presentation of the causes, meaning and variability of Down's syndrome rapidly elided into a consideration of its probability, with the question of the nature of the condition almost immediately backgrounded.

The probability of Down's syndrome

We will now consider the ways in which doctors described the probabilistic component of pre-test risks. Although this might be considered a relatively simple task, close examination demonstrates its complexity, and shows that probabilistic knowledge could be presented to women in many different ways. We have already discussed, in the Introduction, the exclusion of other factors than maternal age from the application of the probability heuristic to the pre-test prediction of Down's syndrome births. This exclusion had the effect of generating an organisationally manageable number of cases, and strengthened the facticity of probabilities based on maternal age. Our discussion will begin with a consideration of another, little discussed complication, namely second-order uncertainty about these maternal age-related probability estimates. We will then explore doctors' accounts of probability during hospital consultations, in relation to the following rather extensive range of complicating issues: the calibration of maternal age; qualitative versus quantitative depictions of probabilities; references to probabilities of genetic abnormalities other than Down's syndrome; changes in the probability of Down's syndrome over the course of the pregnancy; selection of the probability that the abnormalities in question might or might not occur; the framing of probabilities in relation to those associated with younger and older ages; and mistakes in probabilistic reasoning.

Second-order uncertainty about probability estimates

Second-order uncertainty, in the context of inductive probabilistic reasoning, refers to the degree of acknowledged inaccuracy in an incidence estimate (Lehner, Laskey and Dubois, 1996). Accurate estimation of the rate of occurrence of uncommon events in a population requires very large samples. In practice, maternal age-related risks have been assessed through extrapolation from the combined results of a number of smaller studies (Cuckle, Wald and Thompson, 1987) which employed different methodologies. The statistical association between maternal age and the prevalence of Down's syndrome is well established. However, these probabilities would be more accurately represented in terms of ranges indicating the limits of inductive accuracy. Doctors did not usually express a degree of second-order uncertainty about their risk estimates. Two reasons for this lacuna can be suggested. Firstly, they may have accepted average risk estimates unquestioningly. Secondly, they may have wanted to avoid undermining the credibility of their expert advice about probabilities, themselves a confession of partial ignorance.

Second-order uncertainty was occasionally acknowledged in hospital consultations.

> **Doctor:** *At 36 you've probably got a risk in the order of about 1 in 400 of having a baby with Down's Syndrome.* (Charlotte, aged 36, hospital consultation, 12 weeks, [Fallowfield], amniocentesis)

Rapp (1988) detected a form of code-switching, discussed further in the next section, in which genetic counsellors offered rounded, more approximate, representations of probabilities to less educated women. Ironically, these simplified statistics captured the rough and ready status of the cited probabilities better than the spuriously accurate ones.

Doctors more frequently presented maternal age-related risks in a way which suggested their precision. The attachment of significance to the small probability difference discussed in the next quotation was predicated on the implicit assumption that the statistics cited possess sufficient accuracy for it to matter.

> **Doctor:** *You are 36, and for someone who is 36, as you can see from this chart, the age-related risk at 36, you have 1 in 310. Because you are 36 and a bit, it is just a little bit more than that. Now that is about 290.* (Heather, aged 36, hospital consultation [Bell], 16 weeks, no genetic tests)

Although the final risk estimate was qualified by an expression of uncertainty, the context of correcting a probability downwards from 1:310

to 1:290 suggested only a small degree of imprecision in the final figure given. The difference between these two estimates may sound significant. But, for example, in two samples of 10000 in which 1:290 and 1:310 women had babies with Down's syndrome, prevalences of 35 and 32 babies (with rounding to the nearest whole number) would be found. A massive sample of women aged 36 would be required to reliably detect such a difference.

The unusually brisk way in which probability was presented to the younger woman whose consultation is quoted below can be understood in relation to its communication context, with the doctor dismissing serum screening as inappropriate for someone of her age.

> **Doctor:** *You are 27. Your risk for sporadic Down's is 1 in 1210.* (Lucy, aged 27 [Loftus], hospital consultation, 12 weeks, no genetic tests)

Statements of second-order uncertainty may reference a number of sources of doubt (Heyman, Henriksen and Maughan, 1998) including the statistical imprecision of inductive estimates and limited knowledge. (For a person who is completely lost, the probability that turning left rather than right will take him in the correct direction is 50 per cent.) The following quotation refers to the latter, rather than to the unreliability of the underlying probability statistics which doctors drew upon.

> **Doctor:** *Your risk is about 1 in 900, 1 in 1000, probably less because the overall is 1 in 900. Probably your risk is 1 in 1500.* (Ruth, aged 27, hospital consultation [Laughton], 12 weeks, serum screening)

The doctor first cited the approximate probability of Down's syndrome for the local population of pregnant women. The doctor then adjusted this estimate to allow for this woman's relatively young maternal age, but qualified it as 'probable', presumably because the standard maternal age-related table of Down's syndrome probabilities was not to hand.

The term *'probably'* in the next quotation may have been used because the statistics offered by the Northern Genetic Service (1997) stopped at maternal age 45.

> **Doctor:** *You are 46 ... At 45 the risk is 1 in 30, so it is probably 1 in 20 to 1 in 30 at your age.* (Mary, aged 46, hospital consultation [Anderson], 15 weeks, amniocentesis)

The calibration of maternal age

As noted in the Introduction, some confusion was detected about the point in the pregnancy process at which a woman's age should be measured, since her age at conception, at the time of having a test, or at delivery could be used. One doctor measured a woman's age, for risk assessment purposes, with reference to the point in time at which she was tested.

Doctor: *By the age of 36, the risk is about 1 in 310. When you get into the 40s, it starts to increase rapidly.*
Pregnant woman: *What about 37?*
Doctor: *Well this is the age that you have the baby, the age when we would test, so that's what it's done by. So you are 37 now, and you would be having the test whilst you are 37.*
Pregnant woman: *Well I'm 36, but by the time I have it I'll be 37 and a half.*
Doctor: *Well, so it's done on the age of when you have the test.* (Penny, aged 36, hospital consultation [Lewin], 12 weeks, amniocentesis)

Another doctor calibrated a woman's age correctly in relation to the time of delivery.

Doctor: *So you are 40 when the baby is born. Well, they say that the risk of delivering a DS to a 40 year old is 1 in 110.* (Sheila, aged 39, hospital consultation [Bell], 11 weeks, no genetic tests)

The first quotation underestimated the woman's risk of Down's syndrome, 1:240 at the age of 37, rather than the stated 1:310.

It may be objected that, given the imprecision of the underlying risk estimates, such differences should be dismissed as relatively trivial. However, their existence can be used to establish two more general features of doctor/patient risk communication which will be discussed further below. Firstly, doctors themselves were sometimes confused by the complexities of probabilistic reasoning. Secondly, they may have attempted to mount displays of expertise about sometimes difficult issues in order to retain women's confidence.

Quantitative versus qualitative representations of probabilities

Rapp (1988) found that genetic counsellors communicated probabilities in three ways: through qualitative description; by giving rounded numerical statistics; or by giving unrounded statistics. Counsellors appeared to make assumptions about women's educational level and comprehension, offering qualitative descriptions to the least educated and unrounded statistics to the most. We also found these three forms of coding for pre-test probabilities of Down's syndrome. Women were given this statistic, rounded to 10 or less, in 11 of the 16 transcribed consultations, and to 100 in a further two. Qualitative descriptions of risk, for example as *'higher'*, without any quantified probabilities were all that was provided in three consultations. Marteau *et al.* (1994) found, similarly, in a London teaching hospital, that a numerical probability of Down's syndrome was given in 15 out of 21 consultations with obstetricians.

We found evidence in our study that more accurate encoding of pre-test probabilities was one element in a fuller account of the risk picture. Doctors spoke significantly longer (t = 2.2 with 14 d.f., P = 0.05) during consultations in which probabilities were rounded to the nearest 10 (average word count = 1505) than in those in which probabilities were rounded to the nearest 100 or presented qualitatively (average word count = 855).

We were unable to ascertain the educational background of individuals within this sample, and so could not test whether more educated women were given more accurate probability estimates. However, one woman, a research midwife aged 36 married to a University lecturer, mentioned in interview having been cited a probability of 1:311 of having a baby with Down's syndrome. This example suggests that some code switching may have occurred, since none of the sample whose hospital consultations were recorded received statistics coded with this impressive but questionable degree of accuracy.

Several doctors stated that they modified their presentation of the genetic screening/testing decision tree to take account of presumed differences in women's ability to understand complex probabilistic information. The doctor quoted below was concerned to avoid appearing, through use of technical language, to subvert the right of less *'clever'* women to make their own choices about genetic screening/testing.

Doctor: *I think you've got to have an ability where you can sit down with a patient and adjust your little speech according to the type of patient you are confronted with, because in* [catchment area for hospital] *we see a large variety of people. And you can't expect to give a very technical type of talk to, say, a woman who, you know, obviously is maybe intellectually* *not that clever. And you have to have a way of making things easy for her to understand, and not appear to be sitting there and saying, well, you know, not give them the idea that you think this needs to be done, therefore, you should do it; that is, always, do your best to give them knowledge and mental counselling and make the patient feel that you are not deciding. But you still give them views on what the risks and everything are, in language that she can understand* (Rowntree, interview)

However, doctors could not assess women's intelligence, and, at best, could only form stereotypical inductions about their educational or socio-economic level. Moreover, assessment of a woman's comprehension potential could easily be confounded by sub-culturally variable value judgements.

Midwife: *You find that some of them, in the low paid group, they just say, 'Well, it doesn't matter what he comes like, he will be loved and all the rest.' So I don't think they go too much into the thinking side of things when they are having babies. It is more like a biological thing with having a baby. They don't think about the end result, or how they are going to cope afterwards. They get themselves pregnant and then they have it* (Lane, Midwife)

The use of a biological-causal explanation in this account is logically entwined with dismissal of acceptance of Down's syndrome as irrational. However, the perspective which is criticised would be endorsed by the disability movement (Oliver, 1990) and by academic writers who challenge the medicalisation of Down's syndrome (Bailey, 1996). Disagreement about values, in this case perceived rejection of the culture of medicine, can easily be confounded with lack of intelligence, education or foresight.

One piece of qualitative evidence suggests that doctors tended not to provide probabilistic information when they regarded the screening/testing decision as unproblematic. In two of the three consultations in which the doctor did not provide a quantitative pre-test probability of Down's syndrome, the decision was made at the start of the consultation, rather than at its end, as in the other 14 cases. One involved a woman of 39 who opted for amniocentesis at the start of the consultation, and the other a woman of 25 whose hospital doctor ruled out genetic screening/testing as inappropriate. Presumably, the doctor in each case felt that the woman did not need to know her numerical probability of Down's syndrome because the screening/testing decision had already been made, either by her or on her behalf. However, in the third consultation in which a quantitative probability was not offered, with a woman aged 38 who eventually selected serum screening, the decision had not been predetermined. We can offer no explanation of this anomalous case.

Down's syndrome versus genetic abnormalities

Doctors often began their consultations with older women by raising the risk of Down's syndrome as the main topic on the agenda, as noted above. Other, less common genetic conditions which the tests could detect were mentioned in only two consultations. Although Down's syndrome occurs more frequently than any other single chromosomal disorder, the probabilities of these individually rarer conditions add up to a significant total. Moreover, this risk representation excludes consideration of genetic abnormalities which were not currently assessed, for example cystic fibrosis.

One doctor mentioned other abnormalities in the context of the distress which a woman would feel whilst waiting for the results of amniocentesis after positive serum screening.

> **Doctor:** *You have to decide then* [after positive amniocentesis result] *what you are going to do. And it's not only Down's that we are talking about. It's other abnormalities, some less serious, some more serious.* (Heather, aged 36, hospital consultation [Bell], 16 weeks, no genetic tests)

The probability of the baby having one of these other abnormalities was not specified. The woman had decided before the consultation not to be tested because she did not believe in abortion and did not wish to risk receiving a false screen positive. She had not retained any information about chromosomal disorders which, given her concerns, did not interest her.

> **Interviewer:** *Did you talk . . . about Down's Syndrome?*
> **Pregnant woman:** *Vaguely.*
> **Interviewer:** *That is, the reason why they offer it to you at 35?*
> **Pregnant woman:** *Vaguely.* (Heather, aged 36, interview after taped hospital consultation [Bell], 18 weeks, no genetic tests)

Consideration during the consultation of conditions other than Down's syndrome did not, in this context, strengthen the argument for genetic screening/testing, as it did in the consultation discussed below. In this second case, the doctor quantified the probability of a chromosomal abnormality of any kind, not just Down's syndrome.

> **Doctor:** *At 36, the risk to you of having a Down's baby, so that is a chromosome abnormality, the thing that you are no doubt worried about now, is about 1 in 175. About that. The risk of you having a baby with any sort of chromosome problem. I know everyone talks about Down's babies. But there are lots of others, called Edward Syndrome, Potter's Syndrome, Turner Syndrome, lots of different ones, is about 1 in 90, so that is your background risk of a chromosome problem is about 1 in 90 at 36 years old.* (Sarah, aged 36, hospital consultation [Dickson], 10 weeks, amniocentesis)

This widening of scope more or less doubled the probability which the woman was asked to worry about, and may have tilted the balance towards her accepting amniocentesis at a relatively young age for this hospital.

Why did doctors, in general, not discuss these other genetic problems? We may speculate that they did not wish to complicate further the already difficult task of explaining the risks and detection of genetic abnormalities. Such simplification, however, undermined the rationality of the genetic screening/testing enterprise, since women took decisions unaware of most of the genetic risks which they faced. The difference between the 1:90 risk of any chromosome problem, and the 1:175 risk of Down's syndrome which was cited in the above quotation outweighs those which were used to decide on the age threshold for genetic screening.

Changes in probabilities during the course of the pregnancy

As noted in the Introduction, the probability of a woman giving birth to a baby with Down's syndrome and other chromosomal conditions changes during the course of her pregnancy because of the higher than average rate of spontaneous abortion of abnormal foetuses. This additional consideration was mentioned only once in the 16 consultations which we analysed.

> **Doctor:** *So you are 40 when the baby is born. Well, they say that the risk of delivering a DS to a 40 year old is 1 in 110. Now, in fact, the risk*

is, in fact, more than that because of natural wastage. It's more than 1 in 100, in the 90s. It's actually the risk at delivery. (Sheila, aged 39, hospital consultation [Bell], 11 weeks, no genetic tests)

The risk estimates based on regression equations put forward by Cuckle, Wald and Thompson (1987) indicate a probability of $1:110$ of a woman aged 40 at the time of delivery giving birth to a baby with Down's syndrome. This statistic takes account of *'natural wastage'*. Although the quotation is far from clear, the risk *'in the 90s'* which is cited may refer to the probability of Down's syndrome being detected earlier in the pregnancy. A substantial proportion of foetuses with Down's syndrome will be spontaneously aborted between the time of the test and that of birth. Therefore, a higher proportion of women will carry such foetuses at this time than would give birth to a baby with Down's syndrome in the absence of selective abortion. Not surprisingly, most doctors avoided raising yet another complexity, and presented the background probability at birth as an unchanging feature of the pregnancy. This tactic enabled them to avoid undermining the facticity of their risk estimates, as did non-discussion of genetic disorders other than Down's syndrome.

The framing of probabilities

The stories which women were given about the risk of Down's syndrome most commonly represented this probability as a simple, unqualified fact, without reference to the complicating issues discussed above. Nevertheless, the same numerical probability could take on a quite different meaning depending upon the way in which it was framed. We will discuss two such framing effects: firstly, the way in which the seriousness of the risk associated with a given age was scaled in relation to those faced by younger and older women; and, secondly, the direction, positive and/or negative, from which a probability was described.

In 10 of the 13 hospital consultations in which a quantitative pre-test probability of Down's syndrome was cited, the doctor placed this statistic in the context of risks faced by other age-groups, in order to help the woman to interpret its magnitude. With younger women, doctors could use framing information to support the idea that their level of risk did not justify genetic screening/testing.

Doctor: *You are 27. Your risk for sporadic Down's is 1 in 1210. If you were 37, it is 1 in 240. So there is quite a dramatic change in that ten years. And it is really that sort of age group, as I say, about 30s onwards,* *that's the area, that's the age group we target, because, as I say, it is 1 in 1210, it is a pretty low risk at the best of times.* (Lucy, aged 27, hospital consultation [Loftus], 12 weeks, no genetic tests)

Their relative youth limited or precluded use of framing information from below their own age with younger women. However, the doctor quoted below de-emphasised the higher probabilities which older women faced by offering only a qualitative comparison. The doctor also invited the woman to consider the probability of a woman being young, given that her baby had Down's syndrome, as well as the more usual and personally relevant probability, cited later in the consultation, of a woman having Down's syndrome given that she was young. (The distinction between these two types of probability is discussed more fully in the Introduction.)

Doctor: *Although the risk is much lower when you are 27 we know that three-quarters of Down's syndrome babies are actually born to mothers under the age of 34. Now that is not because it is more common under 34 but because most women have their babies under 34.* (Ruth, aged 27, hospital consultation [Laughton], 12 weeks, serum screening)

The combination of qualitative framing and inversion of the personally relevant risk numerator/denominator, albeit with a qualifying explanation, may have contributed to this woman's acceptance of serum screening at a relatively young age.

At the oldest ages, risk could only be framed in relation to younger women, and these comparisons brought out the gravity of the risks which they faced.

Doctor: *You are 46. If you were 15, your risk would be in 1 in 1580. If you were 30, the risk at that age alone is 1 in 910. At 45 the risk is 1 in 30, so it is probably 1 in 20 to 1 in 30 at your age. That still means that the majority of babies don't have Down's syndrome, but that there is what you might regard as quite a significant chance of the baby having Down's syndrome.* (Mary, aged 46, hospital consultation [Anderson], 15 weeks, amniocentesis)

The doctor immediately followed up this warning by raising the issue of genetic testing which the preceding discussion was clearly intended to legitimise.

When advising a woman in the middle of the child-bearing period, the doctor could frame her probability of giving birth to a baby with Down's syndrome in relation to either or both younger and older ages, with varying degrees of emphasis. The resulting messages would, intentionally or unintentionally, communicate a different slant on the magnitude of a woman's risk, particularly about whether it should be categorised as 'high' or 'low'. The framing offered below supported the pre-consultation decision of the woman in question not to undergo genetic screening or testing.

Doctor: *What we also need to discuss is, you are just on the verge of the increasing risk for Down's syndrome. You aren't in a terribly high risk at all. You are 36. And for someone who is 36, as you can see from this chart, the age-related risk at 36, you have 1 in 310 . . . But when you look at a 15 year old, her risk of having a Down's baby is 1 in 1500. The background risk, overall is about 1 in 700. So, you can see, you've probably got a double than average risk. You are still very low. At the age of 45 it goes to 1 in 30, so it's 10 times less than that.* (Heather, age 36, hospital consultation [Bell], 16 weeks, no genetic tests)

The qualitative classification of a risk as 'low' or 'high' entails a value judgement about its seriousness and acceptability (Heyman and Henriksen, 1998b, pp. 86–7). Emphasis on comparison with the oldest group helped to reinforce the relative lowness of the risk this woman faced.

The next quotation conveys a somewhat different interpretation of a similar level of risk, which is defined as *'quite low'* rather than *'very low'*, and is sized in relation to women aged 40 rather than 45.

Doctor: *So that, if I can give you a very approximate figure, women who are 20 have about a 1 in 2000 risk of a Down's syndrome baby, which is perceived as being a low risk. But that's why, now and then, young women do have Down's syndrome babies. When you reach the age of 35, your risk of a Down's syndrome baby is about 1 in 350. It's not 1 in 10, or 1 in 20, but 1 in 350, which is still quite low. When you are 40, it's 1 in 100, all right, so the risk really goes up to around 1 per cent when you are in your later, sort of 30s maybe 40s.* (Susan, aged 35, hospital consultation [Gould], 15 weeks, serum screening)

The contrast between the woman's low risk category and the higher risk faced by older age groups is not so sharply drawn as in the previous quotation. This difference in emphasis may have supported her decision to undergo serum screening.

The doctor quoted below framed the risk of a woman aged 39 only in relation to a younger age group.

> **Doctor:** *Now, at the age of 39, the risk of you having a Down's syndrome baby is getting close to, the percent risk is going to be 1 in 120, 1 in 130 chance . . . Whereas, if you had had a baby when you were 25, the risk then would be something like 1 in 1500. Women who are 25, for every 1 in 1500 women who have a baby, one is likely to have a Down's syndrome baby. So it goes up. What this means now is that for every 125, 130 women at the age of 39 who have a baby, one would be at risk of having a Down's syndrome baby.* (Marietta, aged 39, hospital consultation [Laughton], 10 weeks, amniocentesis)

This presentation served as the introduction to a consideration of screening/testing options, which immediately followed. We may speculate that if the risks faced by women aged 45 had been mentioned, they would have made those affecting a woman of 39 appear relatively low, and so weakened the foundation for the subsequent discussion of screening and testing. A quotation from the interview undertaken after the genetic consultation demonstrates the impact of the framing comparison with younger women.

> **Interviewer:** *Had it been 1200 or something, I would have been saying, 'That's excellent.' But 120 just seems so small [i.e. high] to me. I mean, I know it isn't, but when you say it, I know what you mean, but it just seems small.* (Marietta, aged 39, interview after taped hospital consultation [Laughton], 12 weeks, amniocentesis)

Similarly, the absence of a comparison with older age groups reinforced the categorisation of the woman quoted below, aged 35, as 'borderline' for 'high risk'.

> **Doctor:** *What age were you when you had the last one?*
> **Pregnant woman:** *33*
> **Doctor:** *Right. So, when you were 33, the chances of you having a baby, just by your age alone, you know, if you took a large number of women who are 33 having a baby, it would be 1 in 570. So, if 570 women aged 33 had a baby, one of them by chance would have a baby with Down's Syndrome. At 35 the risks are 1 in 380. Now, why I say I call this the*

borderline, it obviously varies according to what you think is a high risk.
(Margaret, aged 35, hospital consultation [Anderson], 14 weeks, serum screening)

This woman's assessment of the seriousness of the risk she faced was anchored on its one-sided framing.

Interviewer: *Did Dr [name] give you numbers? . . .*
Pregnant woman: Yes. *[The doctor] showed me.*
Interviewer: *How did that make you feel? Did that mean anything to you?*
Pregnant woman: *It made me more aware of the actual risk.* [The doctor] *compared from 32 to 36, you know, the risk that I had when I carried* [previous child] *to now, about three years, and that made me take more notice.* (Margaret, aged 35, interview after taped hospital consultation [Anderson], 16 weeks, serum screening)

As well as being used to define a woman's risk as relatively low, comparisons with the higher risks faced by older women could also be employed to convey the opposite impression.

Doctor: *The age-related risk, risk for Down's is 1 in 310, right? And as you can see, it climbs quite a lot. When are you 37?*
Pregnant woman: *May 3rd.*
Doctor: *Alright. So somewhere between 1 in 310 and 1 in 240.*
Pregnant woman: *Right.*
Doctor: *Compared with a girl of 15, you know, but compared with a girl of 45 it's 1 in 30. It's going to take off.* (Maria, aged 36, hospital consultation [Bell], 11 weeks, serum screening)

This woman could well have concluded that she personally was slipping into a risk abyss. The first part of the quotation suggested that risk increases rapidly at her age, making it necessary to determine her age to the nearest month. The second part did not convey a favourable comparison with the risks faced by older women, but that her own risk was *'going to take off'*. As so often in health risk analysis, the trend within the population, in this case for the prevalence of Down's syndrome to be associated with maternal age, may be confused with processes appertaining to individuals. A comparison with older women which could have reassured, as in the consultation with Susan, discussed above, was turned into an alarming personal projection. The post-consultation interview with Maria supported this interpretation.

Interviewer: *How did that, did you relate to the chart?*
Pregnant woman: *I looked at, well I looked at my age, and I thought, 'Oh I'm up there'. I mean, it went right down to a younger person. And yes, it was good to see that, because, obviously, you are wondering, as you get nearer 40, what the chances are.* (Maria, aged 36, interview after taped hospital consultation [Bell], 15 weeks, serum screening)

It can be concluded that, although the presentation of a woman's own age-related risk was more or less standardised around the statistics supplied by the Northern Genetics Service, the qualitative stance taken towards it was not. Different ways of framing risk in relation to other age groups could reinforce messages about risk acceptability. This conclusion supports the finding of a quantitative study, based on hypothetical vignettes given to psychology students (Shiloh and Sagi, 1989). The results showed that relatively low probabilities of genetic abnormalities appeared lower if comparative data on more probable problems were presented, whilst comparisons with less probable risks made relatively high probability outcomes appear more likely.

Positive versus negative representations of pre-test probabilities

A quantitative probability may be represented in one of two ways, in terms of the chances that an event either will or will not occur. For example, a woman might be told that she has a 1:200 chance of bearing, or a 199:200 chance of not bearing, a baby with Down's syndrome. These two statistically equivalent types of statement may be used to convey different attitudes towards the risk in question. Doctors might offer the second rendition of probability, which highlights the probability that an adverse event will not occur, in an effort to provide reassurance.

Doctor: *Let's talk about 37 year olds. Your age-related risk is 1 in 240. That means effectively, you've got 239 chances out of 240 of not having a baby that has got Down's. Alright?* (Joan, aged 37, hospital consultation [Bell], 11 weeks, amniocentesis)

Within the 13 hospital consultations in which doctors provided women with quantitative pre-test estimates of the probability of Down's syndrome, probabilities were, in each case, presented in the first instance from a negative direction, in terms of the risk of the baby having the condition. In five cases, the doctor also discussed the probability of the woman not having a baby with Down's syndrome. These women were older (mean age = 38.8, N = 5) than those who only received the negative rendition of Down's syndrome risk (mean age = 33.9, N = 8), and the difference was almost statistically significant (t = 2.0 with 11 d.f., P = 0.07, two-tailed test). This finding suggests that doctors used the positive version particularly with older women, whom they classified as being at higher risk and therefore, perhaps, in greater need of reassurance. The following quotation from an interview with a hospital doctor supports this interpretation.

Doctor: *When they come back with their risk assessment, say they've got a one in 40 risk, they face an increased risk of one in 40 of having a baby affected by Down's, then I try and turn it round and say that there are 39 chances out of 40 that everything is okay . . . I try to turn it round, and put it in the positive figure.* (Bell, interview)

In only one case, that of a woman aged 39 who was told only that she faced a risk of about 1:100 of having a baby with Down's syndrome, was the rule that the oldest women would be offered this *'positive figure'* clearly broken. The doctor may have concluded from the determined fashion in which this woman confronted risk that reassurance was not needed.

Doctor: *I gather you are interested in age-related testing. Why is that?*
Pregnant woman: *Because I am 40 this year, and I've heard the older you get the higher your risk of Down's syndrome and spina bifida.* (Sheila, aged 39, hospital consultation [Bell], 11 weeks, no genetic tests)

However, she did not go through with either form of genetic test despite opting for amniocentesis at the hospital consultation. This anomalous finding suggests, at least, that genetic advisers should not underestimate clients' need for reassurance.

Four of the five women who received the second, optimistic rendition of probability were simply offered the reversed statistic, as in the above quotation. However, the oldest woman in our sample, aged 46 was given a qualitative version.

Doctor: *At 45, the risk is 1 in 30, so it is probably 1 in 20 to 1 in 30 at your age. That still means that the majority of babies don't have Down's syndrome, but that there is what you might regard as quite a significant chance of the baby having Down's syndrome.* (Mary, aged 46, hospital consultation [Anderson], 15 weeks, amniocentesis).

Inductively derived probabilities are predicated on a number of implicit assumptions: that the event class in question can be treated as containing homogenous events; that individuals at risk should be categorised in a particular way; and that aggregate properties of categories (e.g. pregnant women of a given age) can be attributed to individuals. The probabilities manufactured through complex cultural, cognitive and empirical processes can be communicated in surprisingly varied ways, so that the same statistic can be given many different meanings.

7
The Hospital Consultation II: Risk and Genetic Screening/Testing

Introduction

In Chapter 6, we explored the complex issues which doctors had to tackle when they discussed genetic risks in hospital consultations. Having discussed these pre-test probabilities, doctors attempted to guide women through the process of decision-making about genetic tests. Our consideration of the further complications which ensued will highlight two central features. Firstly, genetic screening/testing was associated with new risks, over and above those it was designed to prevent, namely emotional distress during the waiting period, miscarriage as a result of amniocentesis and the trauma of abortion. Secondly, the probability of a genetic abnormality could be changed as a result of screening/testing. This second complication arises because probabilities encode limited knowledge about, rather than events in, the natural world, as argued in the Introduction and Chapter 4.

In this chapter, we will first consider communication about the genetic screening/testing decision tree which women had to navigate. We will then discuss communication in the hospital consultation about each of the main screening/testing options on offer, namely, serum screening and amniocentesis. Finally, we will consider communication about the decisions which women actually made, with reference to the issues of choice and decision timing.

Communication about the genetic decision tree

In order to advise women who were considering genetic screening/ testing, doctors had to portray not only the specific options available, but also the general nature of the decision tree which women were required to navigate. We have already discussed one feature of overall decision-making, that women might or might not be required to make prior commitments before finding out their test results (see *'Predicting Future Intentions'* in Chapter 5). In this section, we will discuss three further aspects: the representation of the genetic screening/testing decision tree; the discussion of choice in the hospital consultation; and the sharing, or, more commonly, non-sharing, of responsibility for decision-making between women and partners.

Representation of the genetic screening/testing decision tree

The choices which women were asked to confront in the hospital site for our research are set out in Figure 3.1. This decision tree, as noted in the Introduction, can be thought of as an upwards risk escalator (Heyman and Henriksen, 1998b, pp. 95–103) which women might step onto if they were offered genetic screening/testing, and which they could exit at various points, depending upon test outcomes and their responses to them. Those who test positive at the serum screening and/or amniocentesis stage may find it harder to exit from the risk escalator than if they had not stepped onto it in the first place.

The decision-making process has been considered in Chapters 4 and 5. In this section, we will explore the ways in which this decision tree was presented to women in the hospital consultation. Important variations which may well have affected decision-making will be identified. Women might or might not be told that they should not embark on genetic screening/testing unless prepared to go through with an abortion, or that they should not opt for serum screening unless prepared to live with the risk remaining after a negative result. The screening/testing menus which women were explicitly offered varied substantially.

Women were mostly not given a full description of the screening/testing decision tree set out in Figure 3.1, perhaps because of its complexity. The most complete account observed in the hospital consultations is quoted, almost in full, below.

Doctor: *From that point of view* [maternal age-related genetic risks] *there are various options you can go for. The first, you can do nothing at all. I'll come back to that one. The second option is to have a blood test. The blood test is done at 16 weeks. The blood test is not an infallible test, but it does detect 60–70 per cent of those women who would be at risk of having a Down's syndrome baby. Now it's not a specific test. So, not only* *are there sometimes babies missed by it, but all the test is, it gives you an increased risk of having a Down's Syndrome baby. And if the test shows that you are at an increased risk, what we would offer to do a week later is an amniocentesis test; an amniocentesis test being where we take some fluid from around the baby, the cells of the baby are then cultured in a laboratory, and then, three weeks later, we get a result back which tells us the sex of the baby, if you wish to know. It tells us whether the baby has Down's syndrome, and it tells us about a few other abnormalities. As I'm sure you are aware, . . . the amniocentesis does carry a risk. And no matter how expert or careful we are at doing the amniocentesis, between 1 in 100 and 1 in 200 babies are lost as a result of the test . . . Provided the test goes, is uncomplicated, we will not get the results of that test until you are around 19 or 20 weeks pregnant. And we would then, at that point, if you had a Down's syndrome baby, offer to terminate the pregnancy . . . Now I often think in terms of what you decide to do. It's better to work from that end backwards. And the questions you have to ask yourself are, 'How do I feel about having a Down's syndrome baby?'.*

Pregnant woman: *I don't want that.*

Doctor: *That's an important question to ask. The second question is, 'Would I be able to go through with the termination of pregnancy?'. Thirdly, how might, still going backwards, how might I feel about losing the baby, a normal baby, having had an amniocentesis test?*

Pregnant woman: *I would be very upset, very.*

Doctor: *You are obviously going to cope if the baby had Down's syndrome, and, again, that is, losing the baby if the baby may have been normal. And then, going back further, if I had just the blood test, how would I feel if the test, hopefully, reassured me that everything was okay, and I subsequently delivered a Down's Syndrome baby?* (Marietta, aged 39, hospital consultation [Laughton], 10 weeks, amniocentesis)

This quotation, from which only a few detailed explanations have been omitted, sets out with unusual clarity and explicitness the complexity of the decision maze which women were asked to navigate. However, even this exposition does not provide an uncontroversial picture of the choices women had to make. The very low probability of a screen negative given that the foetus has Down's syndrome (see the Introduction) is discussed, whilst the much higher probability of a screen positive given that the foetus does not have Down's syndrome is not mentioned. The idea of thinking backwards from an imagined future point in the decision trajectory implies that women who had ruled out termination should select the *'do nothing'* option. As we have seen in Chapter 5 (see the section on *'Time Management'*), women might select genetic screening/testing simply to obtain advance information, or, hopefully, reassurance, or adopt a step-by-step approach to their decisions because they could not anticipate how they would feel after receiving a test result.

Not surprisingly, women could be daunted by the prospect of navigating this complex decision space, and be tempted by the alternative of allowing nature to take its course.

Pregnant woman: *Should you be tempting fate? Should you be messing with what is going on? But I think, ultimately, it is a difficult choice, you know. Is it better not to know anything – ignorance is bliss? Is it better not to know anything, and just go through blindly and naively? Or is it better to be faced with all the choices and scientific blurb which confuses you and baffles you even further?* It is very difficult (Charlotte, aged 36, interview after taped hospital consultation [Fallowfield], amniocentesis)

Erosion of the right not to know resulting from pressure to be genetically responsible has also been noted in relation to the screening of women for breast cancer risk (Hallowell, 1999).

Other women welcomed the prospect of increased control over the future which the genetic screening/testing system provided.

Pregnant woman: *I am the type that would rather know and do something about it. I am not one to leave everything to fate. I think you have got a lot of control over it. I mean technology has moved forward from when my mother had children.* (Joan, aged 37, interview after taped hospital consultation [Bell], 11 weeks, amniocentesis)

The above two quotations illustrate contrasting attitudes to fate, respectively as a being which may be 'tempted', and as a future which need not be passively accepted. The former is predicated on a personalistic cosmology (Davison, Frankel and Davey Smith, 1992; Heyman and Henriksen, 1998b, pp. 82–4), based on the belief that the future is managed by a sentient agency. The second woman believed that the future should be actively colonised (Giddens, 1991, p. 111). Navigation of the genetic screening/testing decision tree entailed embracing this perspective, which women accepted with varying degrees of enthusiasm.

The menus presented to women who were offered genetic screening/testing were usually set out in much less detail than in the consultation quoted at the start of this section, and with variable sets of options. One woman was offered chorionic villus sampling as well as the standard serum screening and amniocentesis. The test was available at a regional hospital, but was not provided at the hospital site for our research. Since most women were not told about this possibility, they could not consider it, and were effectively denied an option which is widely used elsewhere. The option of doing nothing, pointed out explicitly in the last quotation was not mentioned in the set of choices offered to a slightly younger woman.

> **Doctor:** *You're 38, so you are wondering about the question of Down's syndrome.*
> **Pregnant woman:** *Yes.*
> **Doctor:** *Have you read anything about DS yet?*
> **Pregnant woman:** *No, just what was in the booklet.*
> **Doctor:** *I think there are two ways we can look at what we are going to do about* [Down's syndrome]. *There is the blood test. What the BT does, it tells you if you are at high risk or at low risk . . . Alternatively, we can go straight to taking some fluid away from around the baby.* (Hazel, aged 38, hospital consultation [Crabtree], 8 weeks, serum screening)

The opening of this consultation is predicated on the doctor's assumption that a woman of 38 would want to actively *'do'* something about the risk of Down's syndrome. Its non-mention excluded the do nothing option from the discussion.

Negotiation of choice

Doctors, in general, adopted a 'liberal' approach to expertise (Heyman and Henriksen, 1998a, pp. 58–9), based on the implicit assumption that they provided the facts about probability whilst women made value judgements about the adversity of Down's syndrome, miscarriage or living with unreduced uncertainty until the baby was born.

> **Doctor:** *I never make the decision, never. And I will say to them that we are offering them advice and choice, but they will make the decision, and that they will have to play God and doctor and parent, and we don't do that. And if they make a bad decision, they have to live with that, not me. I walk away from it.* (Laughton, interview)

For this reason, doctors sometimes withheld advice about the decision itself even when it was requested.

Pregnant woman: *I would have the blood test, I think. I have dis-*
cussed it with my, I mean would you – what do you advise? It's just, I
don't know what to do.
Doctor: *It's something you have to discuss at home, and then you make*
an informed decision between you. Whatever you do is right. We will go
along with it, but it has to be you. (Maria, aged 36 [Bell], hospital consultation, 11 weeks, serum screening)

However, this message was interpreted by the above pregnant woman
as indicating medical ignorance rather than liberalism.

Pregnant woman: *And then you have to decide what you want to*
do. I mean it's your decision isn't it? Nobody can decide it for you. Because
I was asking Dr [Bell] what should I do. [The doctor] said, 'I don't
know.' And, I mean, my husband doesn't know a lot about it, he doesn't.
But I've had the information and the sheet, and he didn't read it, but, I
mean, I can appreciate that. He doesn't really understand. (Maria, aged
36, interview after taped hospital consultation [Bell], 15 weeks, serum
screening)

The above respondent, perhaps, did not fully understand the distinction, itself problematic, between facts and values on which the doctor's
refusal to give advice was based. She recalled that the doctor had said,
'*I don't know*' in response to her request for advice. His ignorance is
described in the same terms as that of her husband who had not bothered to read the information leaflet. But the transcript of the hospital
consultation, quoted above, shows that the doctor had not confessed
ignorance, but had suggested that only she and her family could make
an informed choice. This surface error may result from a good understanding of the culture of medicine, however, since doctors tend to
offer options when they believe that a treatment of choice cannot be
definitively prescribed (Silverman, 1987, pp. 146–8). The pregnant
woman was left with an existential burden of choice which her husband
would not share with her. Lippman-Hand and Fraser (1979b) also found
that some parents sought their counsellor's advice about the genetic
test decision they ought to take despite the non-directive stance of
counselling ideology.

Whilst the last woman quoted sought concrete advice about which
decision to take, others appreciated their doctor's attempt to separate
facts from values.

Pregnant woman: [The doctor was] *very neutral, I thought, very business-like.* [The doctor's] *personality, which is what I liked, didn't come into it.* [The doctor] *was saying the things that needed to be said without any sort of judgement . . .* [The doctor] *had all the facts there, all the facts were there, but it was still my choice* (Joan, aged 37, interview after taped hospital consultation [Bell], 11 weeks, amniocentesis)

Even when doctors did offer concrete advice about the appropriateness of a test, they sometimes pulled back from making a specific recommendation.

Doctor: *The blood test is really a test that was designed to screen younger women, because most of the babies have been had to women in their 20's, and things like that. We were looking for a test that would identify those younger women that were at higher risk than average of having a baby with Down's syndrome. So it isn't quite as applicable to ladies of your age as it is to younger people.*
Pregnant woman: *Right . . . Would you then say that it's not worth having the blood test, go straight to the amnio if that's what you would decide?*
Doctor: *Well I wouldn't quite know that, but you are probably right. The other side of that is, when we do the tests, and if it shows that it has a higher than average risk, we still have to do an amniocentesis to make the diagnosis.* (Charlotte, aged 36, hospital consultation [Fallowfield], 12 weeks, amniocentesis)

The suggestion to the pregnant woman that *'you are probably right'* relocates the judgement about test appropriateness firmly with her, even though the doctor initially mentioned the unsuitability of serum screening. However, this firm recommendation of amniocentesis at a relatively young age did match her own views.

Interviewer: *Can you remember what* [hospital doctor] *said to you?*
Pregnant woman: *Yes, I think so, more or less.* [The doctor] *more or less said that if, if you have a blood test, you will come up as 400, 400 to 1 I think* [the doctor] *said, that will be your figure, and the risk of miscarriage is 200 to 1. Make your own decisions from that. But if I think, if I remember rightly,* [the doctor] *said, 'If I was you, I would have it', which was what I wanted* [the doctor] *to say.* (Charlotte, aged 36, interview after taped hospital consultation [Fallowfield], 16 weeks, amniocentesis)

As with Maria, quoted above, the recall error in the above quotation resulted from a sensible interpretation of what was said. The doctor did not directly advise the woman to choose amniocentesis, but implicitly recommended this course of action. Doctors who attempted to *'walk away'* from decision-making placed on themselves the unattainable requirement to offer neutral, value-free advice, as one doctor acknowledged.

Doctor: *You try to give them non-directional counselling if you can, although I don't think any of us give non-directional counselling.* (Fallowfield, interview)

We have seen, in Chapter 6, that even the apparently simple task of communicating probabilities allowed many different slants to be put onto the evidence. Midwives, who would deal with a number of registrars and consultants, directly experienced, and were more likely than doctors to recognise, differences of medical opinion.

Pregnant midwife: *Mr _____* [hospital doctor] *doesn't like serum screenings at all, so* [this doctor] *would prefer for them not to have them, and go directly for amnios if they needed to. Mr _____* [second hospital doctor] *doesn't.* [The second doctor] *tends to try and persuade them to have screening.* (Shirley, midwife, aged 34, interview, 20 weeks, no genetic tests)

We have argued (Heyman and Henriksen, 1998a, pp. 59–61) that genuine power-sharing between health professionals and service users requires the former to recognise the inescapable subjectivity in which their expertise is embedded.

Family decision-making

Women faced with life or death responsibility for the genetic future of their baby had to negotiate the role of their partners in the decision-making process. Several women felt that they had been left to make the decision alone, but that their husband was willing to support them in whatever choice they took.

Pregnant woman: *He* [husband] *said, 'Well, I'm 100 per cent with whatever you decide.'* (Margaret, aged 35, interview after taped hospital consultation [Anderson], 16 weeks, serum screening)

The allocation of responsibility to women can be easily explained in terms of the application of traditional sex roles to the novel, esoteric activity of genetic risk management, with women held responsible for 'quality control' of foetuses and children (Rapp, 1999, p. 87). This juxtaposition of old and new could cause considerable anguish even when a woman felt supported by her partner.

> **Pregnant woman:** *I think it* [decision about genetic screening/testing] *is one of the hardest I've ever had to make really* (Margaret, aged 35, interview after taped hospital consultation [Anderson], 14 weeks, serum screening)

Only one respondent indicated that her husband had participated actively in a joint decision.

> **Pregnant woman:** *So there is no way I could have made the decision on my own.* (Marietta, aged 39, interview after taped hospital consultation [Laughton], 12 weeks, amniocentesis)

Another woman felt that her husband had taken over decision-making, in effect placing himself in charge of the pregnancy.

> **Pregnant women:** *It is more his baby than mine. Yes, at the moment, it is more his baby, isn't it?* (Mary, aged 46, interview after taped hospital consultation [Anderson], 16 weeks, amniocentesis)

A doctor expressed concern that partners might take over decision-making from the pregnant woman.

> **Doctor:** *What irks me a little bit sometimes is if the partner does the answering for the couple. And that is what upsets me, because he is not the one who has to make the final decision, or who has to live with the consequences as much as the girls have* (Bell, interview)

As the above examples show, the management of power-sharing between doctor and pregnant woman intersected with its negotiation between mother and father in ways which could reinforce a woman's sense of facing difficult decisions alone, generate the sharing of parental responsibility, or substitute partner for medical dominance.

Communicating the risk picture after serum screening

Having portrayed a woman's pre-screening risk, in relation to maternal age, doctors attempted to explain how this risk picture would be changed if she decided to undergo serum screening. As noted in the Introduction, the screening procedure in practice at the time of the research (Northern Region Genetics Service, 1995) entailed calculating a risk estimate based on the combination of a woman's age and the results of serum screening. Women whose overall probability of giving birth to a baby with Down's syndrome was estimated to be less than 1:200 were told that they were at low risk. Above this level, women were given a numerical estimate of their risk. This limitation to the risk information they would receive was not explained to women unless they asked.

> **Pregnant woman:** *Do you get to know what* [probability of Down's syndrome] *you come out at?*
> **Doctor:** *No. You know your risk is less than 1 in 200.*
> **Pregnant woman:** *But you are not told?*
> **Doctor:** *You're not told, you are just put at low risk.* (Joan, aged 37, hospital consultation [Bell], 11 weeks, amniocentesis)

In this section, we will explore two issues which doctors attempted to discuss with women during the hospital consultation: the change in a woman's probability of giving birth to a baby with Down's syndrome which would result from serum screening; and the probability of false negatives versus false positives.

The effect of serum screening on probability

The induction of probabilities from observed frequencies entails heuristic acceptance of the ecological fallacy, and attribution of aggregate properties of constructed risk categories to the individuals within them, as argued in the Introduction. However, the tendency of doctors to view probabilities as a natural property of individuals, comparable to a medical condition, rather than as a description of predictive power, sometimes obscured their derivation from constructed risk categories.

Doctor: *When you reach the age of 35, your risk of a Down's syndrome baby is about one in 350 . . . Now that's for all women. So, what I can't tell you at the moment is what your individual risk is . . . In 350 women, only one of them will have a Down's syndrome baby. What the blood test will do is measure hormone levels. And it will give you an individual risk, right. So it will say, it won't tell you that your baby has got Down's syndrome, or hasn't got Down's syndrome . . . But what it does is, instead of giving you the risk of all women who are 35, it gives you your own risk.* (Susan, aged 35, hospital consultation [Gould], 15 weeks, serum screening)

The above doctor distinguished between a collective risk for *'all women who are 35'* and a woman's *'individual risk'*, determined by serum screening. But this test provides no more than an additional way of differentiating women into categories with higher and lower rates of Down's syndrome. The probabilities which the doctor cited are based on cross-classifying women in terms of the combination of maternal age and serum screening results. They do not provide estimates of individual risk, merely a more finely grained sub-classification of cases. The notion of individual risk can be dismissed as an oxymoron. Individual women were either carrying or not carrying babies with Down's syndrome. Probability, in the sense of an expectation about the future (Shafer, 1990) based on induction from observed frequencies, can only reference collectives, however defined. But women, and the doctors who tried to advise and reassure them, were concerned with their individual outcomes, not average statistics. This tension between concern for personal biography and the inherent limitations of aggregate knowledge may have caused some doctors to sometimes exaggerate the power of their knowledge base. In contrast, the representation of the post-serum screening probability as simply *'more accurate'* in the following quotation acknowledged the tentative status of inductive estimates.

Doctor: *The blood test shows a risk of Down's syndrome. It doesn't tell you whether the baby has got it or not, but it gives a more accurate assessment of your risk than just going by your age alone. So, if we took a blood test on every women who was 33, we would, instead of saying that the risk of having a baby with a problem was 1 in 570, we would pick out 1 in 100 of them as being at risk by the blood test.* (Penny, aged 36, hospital consultation [Lewin], 12 weeks, amniocentesis)

Even this representation implies that, with sufficient scientific refinement, a fully accurate probability could be measured. However, full accuracy entails correct prediction, almost achieved through amniocentesis, and the removal of uncertainty. In this circumstance, the probability of giving birth to a baby with Down's syndrome would be either 1 or 0, and risk analysis would not be required. The quotation externalises uncertainty onto individuals, and so maintains the cultural status of risk as a natural entity.

False negatives and positives

The probabilities of false positives and negatives following serum screening were discussed in the Introduction. Strictly speaking, as pointed out, these terms should not be used because 'positive' and 'negative' results only tell a woman that she is at higher or lower risk than the average for her age group. Women who screen 'negative' can give birth to babies with Down's syndrome, whilst most women who screen 'positive' will not give birth to a baby with this condition.

The system for estimating women's probability of giving birth to a baby with Down's syndrome used by the Northern Genetics Service (1995) utilised maternal age as well as serum screening results. Such a system leads to an increased rate of false positives, and a correspondingly reduced rate of false negatives, among older women, as discussed in the Introduction. This complication was not explained to any of the 16 women whose hospital consultations were transcribed. Nor were they told that the balance between the risk of false positives and false negatives depended upon the boundary which the processing laboratory selected for dividing higher and lower risks (1:200 in this case). Even this simplification left doctors with the complex task of delving into Bayesian probabilistic reasoning. As will be shown below, doctors, in general, prioritised prevention of false negatives over avoidance of false positives.

The possibility that serum screening results and pregnancy outcome might not match, in the limited sense discussed above, was mentioned in all but three of the 16 taped hospital consultations. These three consultations involved the oldest women, aged 46, with whom serum screening was not discussed, and two of the youngest women, aged 25 and 27, who were advised not to bother with any form of genetic screening/testing. In the other 13 consultations, the doctor explicitly mentioned the risk of false negatives, but the risk of false positives was discussed in only five of the 16 consultations. Hence, in eight consultations, only false negatives, and not false positives, were considered.

In just one case, that of the woman aged 27 referred to above, the doctor mentioned the risk of false positives, but not negatives, in a context of suggesting the inappropriateness of serum screening.

> **Doctor:** *But if you have a blood test screening, as I say, it can start you on, on the track for a fair amount of heartache, in terms of problems with your results, interpretation of the results. It might* [come back with] *a relatively high value, or an abnormal value in relation to, and if that was the case, then we would obviously have to talk in terms of amniocentesis because, whatever you have read or heard about blood tests, screening is only screening* (Ruth, aged 27, hospital consultation [Laughton], 12 weeks, no genetic tests)

The hypothesis that doctors advising women deemed to be at higher risk of a Down's syndrome birth on account of their age prioritised the risk of false negatives over the risk of false positives is supported by the following quotation.

> **Doctor:** *False positives don't worry me as much because, even though I have never actually lost a baby related to an amniocentesis yet. And so, for people who have passed the learning curve, it is possible that the foetal loss rate is smaller than the quoted risk. But the false negatives worry me. And certainly there was a false negative at* [nearby hospital] *which I know the lady was, had a Down's baby, and she made inquiries about legal action against the hospital. Now that, I mean the legal aspect, doesn't worry me, but the impact worries me . . . It is such a big thing to take on. And until we can get the false negative rate down, I think I would rather not offer it to everybody, because it isn't perfect.* (Bell, interview)

This argument focuses on the harm caused by rare false negatives, whilst discounting the negative impact of a much more probable false positive. The same doctor attributed women's anxiety about screen positives to a deficit in their understanding.

> **Doctor:** *I would prefer to give you the results* [of serum screening] *myself because people who screen positive always think that they have got an abnormal pregnancy. They can't see that it's just a blood test.* (Maria, aged 36, hospital consultation [Bell], 11 weeks, serum screening)

This doctor was attempting to avoid confusion between the notions of a 'higher risk' and a 'positive' result, against which counselling has been recommended as a preventative measure (Green, 1994). The attribution of blindness to pregnant women who worry about screen positives suggests that the doctor found it difficult to acknowledge the distress caused by placing women in the higher risk category.

The risk which doctors most emphasised, that of a woman who screened negative giving birth to a baby with Down's syndrome (a Down's syndrome birth, given a negative serum screening result), was the least likely to occur (see Table 0.2), as acknowledged in the following quotation.

> **Doctor:** *I told you that your risk is about 1 in 90 of any abnormality. If your risk comes back, say, 1 in 2500, which is like mid 20s, so, most probably, the baby will be normal. However, if you are the 1 in 2500, and the baby is abnormal, the test won't have been much use for you. That is the big drawback.* (Sarah, aged 36, hospital consultation [Dickson], 10 weeks, amniocentesis)

In contrast, the next quotation refers to the much higher probability that serum screening will not detect a baby with Down's syndrome (of a negative serum screening result, given Down's syndrome).

> **Doctor:** *But you have to remember it still only picks up, at best, 70 per cent of Down's babies. So you do run that risk of 30 per cent, but you have reduced your risk considerably, but not to nil. Some people, even at 37, would opt directly for the amniocentesis. And, again, there is a choice.* (Joan, aged 37, hospital consultation [Bell], 11 weeks, amniocentesis)

Women unfamiliar with the distinction between the probability of A, given B, and the probability of B, given A, could all too easily assume that, as the quotation suggests, they personally faced a 30 per cent probability that serum screening would not detect Down's syndrome. The follow-up interview with the woman whose hospital consultation is quoted above suggests that she had tentatively drawn this conclusion. She asked the midwife interviewer for clarification.

> **Pregnant woman:** *The blood test only picks up 70 per cent, doesn't it?*
> **Interviewer:** *It tells you whether you are at high or low risk.*
> **Pregnant woman:** *That's all. So you could come out low risk, but you could still* [have a baby with Down's syndrome]. (Charlotte, aged 36, interview after taped hospital consultation [Fallowfield], amniocentesis)

However, the statistic cited only applies to the very small sub-set of pregnant women who give birth to a baby with the condition. The above woman, if she tested negative, faced only the much smaller probability of Down's syndrome given a low risk serum screening result. This confusion about a difficult distinction was triggered by the doctor's representation of the false negative probability, and clearly influenced the above woman's selection of amniocentesis at a relatively young age.

The representation of false positives in the five interviews in which this was discussed is illustrated in the following quotation.

> **Doctor:** *Do a lot of women go through a positive* [serum] *test? Do they what we call screen positive? Yes, they do. If we have a look at 37-year-old women here, well 37-year-old women have an age-related risk of 1 in 240. So 239 out of 240 chances are OK, but 1 in 5 will be placed at high risk, 1 in 5, that's 20 per cent. So a lot of women have been worried, and when your age-related risk is still only 1 in 240.* (Joan, aged 37, hospital consultation [Bell], 11 weeks, amniocentesis)

This quotation referred to both versions of the false positive rate shown in Table 0.2, although only one, the probability that a woman will be classified as at higher risk even though the foetus does not have Down's syndrome, was more or less fully worked out. The probability cited (20 per cent) increases with maternal age (Northern Genetics Service, 1998) and varies between hospitals, as noted in the Introduction. Quantification of the probability that a woman aged 37 who screens positive will give birth to a baby with Down's syndrome, $1:48$ on the figures given, as explained in the Introduction, would have highlighted a severe limitation of current screening technology.

However false positive statistics are calculated, they do highlight a major limitation of current screening methods. The above quoted doctor attempted to draw the following comfort from this shortcoming.

> **Doctor:** *Now we will take that one step further. The blood test is only a screen test. It is not a bad risk, four out of five chances of things being alright even if screened positive, 80 per cent chance that things will be OK.* (Joan, aged 37 [Bell], hospital consultation, 11 weeks, amniocentesis)

Women may not find such statistics reassuring. Moreover, as just demonstrated, women of 37 who screened positive, according to this doctor's own figures, faced a 98 per cent probability of not giving birth to a baby with Down's syndrome. In the majority of consultations (11 out of 16), the doctor avoided the topic of false positives entirely, as already noted. But women who were considering their genetic screening/testing options could not make fully informed choices unless they understood the implications of both a lower and a higher risk screening verdict. Such understanding required a grasp of the complexities of probabilistic reasoning which even confused hospital doctors.

Communicating the risk picture after amniocentesis

The doctor discussed amniocentesis, however briefly, in all of the 16 recorded hospital consultations. Some variation in the maternal age boundary below which amniocentesis was considered inappropriate occurred. Five of the youngest women, including two aged 35 and 36, were advised against the test, on the grounds that the risk of inducing a miscarriage was greater than that of detecting a foetus with Down's syndrome.

> **Doctor:** *Now the risk of actually having the test done is somewhere between 1 in 100 and 1 in 200 of women having amniocentesis having a miscarriage because of having the test. And that miscarriage is, well, the chance of having a child with Down's syndrome is only 1 in 570. The chance of having a miscarriage would then be greater than having a child with an abnormality, so you would be more likely to miscarry a perfectly normal baby because of having the test.* (Penny, aged 36, hospital consultation [Lewin], 12 weeks, amniocentesis)

The doctor's advice may have persuaded the above woman, who excluded amniocentesis at the consultation, but she eventually selected this option. The other 11 women, the youngest of whom was aged 35, were offered amniocentesis as a sensible option.

Doctors who offered a risk picture of amniocentesis covered some or all of the following issues: the risk of miscarriage; the balance between this risk and the risk of Down's syndrome; the possibility of errors; the anxiety which women would feel during the wait of up to three weeks for amniocentesis results; and the emotional meaning of termination. However, significant variation in the presentation of these issues could be detected.

The risk of amniocentesis inducing a miscarriage

The risk of miscarriage associated with amniocentesis was sometimes presented as a natural, unalterable fact of nature, and at other times as a byproduct of a human action, namely the performing surgeon's level of skill. Both the probability cited, and the degree of second-order uncertainty attached, differed to some extent. The last quotation represented this value as somewhere between 1:100 and 1:200, whilst the doctor cited below attached a degree of precision to the statistics provided, although the figure of 1:200 is qualified as *'about'*.

> **Doctor:** *The risks of miscarriage from an amnio are about 0.5 per cent, so about 1 in 200 will miscarry, so that is your risk from that.* (Sarah, aged 36 [Dickson], hospital consultation, 10 weeks, amniocentesis)

This doctor's coda of *'that is your risk from that'* conveyed its inescapable facticity.

Other doctors presented the risk of miscarriage not as an invariable feature of the natural world, but as dependent upon the skills of the doctor administering the test.

> **Doctor:** *Amniocentesis, isn't quite as safe* [as serum screening]. *I mean the national figure of losing the baby is 1 in 200, right. So that's, the risk of losing it is half, probably less. But this hospital hasn't lost any in ages. We are all past our learning curve.* (Sheila, aged 39, hospital consultation [Bell], 11 weeks, no genetic tests)

One doctor pointed out the difficulty arising from this reassuring conclusion, that reliable estimates of low probabilities require large samples.

> **Doctor:** *By the statistics, our local risk is probably a hell of a lot less than that. None of us, as far as we know, have lost a baby, related to the test* [amniocentesis]. *That's after many hundred. But, for me, it would only take 4 or 5. I can't remember how many hundreds and hundreds and hundreds I've done, but it would probably only take 4 or 5. But it's probably less than 1 in 200 of losing the baby.* (Maria, aged 36, hospital consultation [Bell], 11 weeks, serum screening)

Whether presented as inherently random or as dependent on the doctor's skill and experience, the miscarriage risk associated with amniocentesis could be discussed in isolation, or related to the overall probability of this adverse event. The latter course was taken in only one hospital consultation.

Doctor: *The downside of amniocentesis is that, first of all, there is a risk. It is difficult to quantify the risk. It used to be said that it was in the order of about 1 per cent, meaning by that that it was 1 per cent above whatever is the risk of miscarriage for your age group. I say, 'whatever is' because, really, we do not know. In round figure terms, we would say 10 per cent possibly. It might even be higher than that, in terms of the actual risk of miscarriage which is inherent in the fact that you are pregnant, and that is something that nobody has control over. So you are adding about roughly 1 per cent to that. In fact, I would say that it is probably less than 1 per cent.* (Linda, aged 39 [Loftus], hospital consultation, 12 weeks, amniocentesis)

By putting the additional risk in an overall context, the doctor made it appear less significant, since amniocentesis was stated to cause an increase in the probability of miscarriage from 10 per cent to less than 11 per cent. The provision of this context may have contributed to the woman's selection of amniocentesis.

Pregnant woman: *Although the test itself has got an extra 1 per cent risk of miscarriage, I would be fairly confident of the test itself.* (Linda, aged 39, interview after taped hospital consultation [Loftus], 14 weeks, amniocentesis)

Balancing the risks of miscarriage and Down's syndrome

Women who wished to avoid the birth of a baby with Down's syndrome had to weigh this risk against that of miscarriage. The balance struck usually took into account maternal age because of its association with the risk of Down's syndrome, as in the next quotation.

Doctor: *We don't routinely offer it to people under 37, because 37 is about the same risk as having an amniocentesis miscarriage as having a baby with Down's syndrome. And we routinely offer it to people above that age because they have a higher risk of having a Down's baby than a miscarriage. Below that, because the risk is about the same, 36/37, we leave it up to you. If you are under 35, then we don't usually raise the spectre of having amniocentesis unless you are very desperate to know.* (Charlotte, aged 36 [Fallowfield], hospital consultation, amniocentesis)

A given probability of two incommensurable outcomes, in this case the birth of a baby with Down's syndrome and a miscarriage, only generates the equal amount of negative utility if these outcomes are assigned the same value. The arbitrariness of this assumption of value equivalence is illustrated in the next quotation.

> **Doctor:** *In my personal view, I can only say if you wanted to do it* [amniocentesis], *then once it gets to being about the same risk or greater, but if it's less, sort of, then you would have twice as much chance of causing a problem with the amniocentesis as it would actually having a baby with a problem. But it depends on how you feel about it, and about this pregnancy, given the fact that it was a surprise in the first place. And that sometimes doesn't make you not want it. Sometimes it makes you want it more.* (Margaret, aged 35, hospital consultation [Anderson], 14 weeks, serum screening)

Although an odds ratio of the probability of a miscarriage divided by that of a Down's syndrome birth was proposed in this consultation, it was then undermined by the acknowledgement of value incommensurability. The more highly a woman values her pregnancy, the lower will be the risk, *ceteris paribus*, of miscarriage which she will be prepared to accept in order to prevent the birth of a baby with Down's syndrome. We have repeatedly emphasised the problematic status of the evidence that amniocentesis causes miscarriages. Women and doctors drew upon the conventional wisdom about this risk.

Donnenfeld (1995) has argued that the cut-off maternal age of 35 for being offered amniocentesis was originally selected because it generated a number of cases which matched the capacity, at the time of their introduction, of laboratories to process tests. If the level of acceptable risk had been set lower, laboratories would have been swamped, whilst a higher cut-off would have left them underemployed. The assumption of value equivalence between miscarriages and Down's syndrome births thus provided a means of legitimating a resource-driven distinction. The only maternal age-related risk statistics available in the early 1970s were grouped into five-year periods. One-year statistics might not have justified setting the cut-off for amniocentesis at the maternal age of 35 years. However, once established, this dividing line became legally enforceable as women in the USA (and the UK) successfully sued on the grounds that they had given birth to a child with Down's syndrome after the age of 35, but had not been offered screening/testing.

Amniocentesis errors

Women who opted for amniocentesis accepted a reportedly greater risk of miscarriage, and the unpleasantness of a needle insertion into the uterus, in order to escape from the uncertainty associated with serum screening. They could not escape this uncertainty entirely, however. Amniocentesis, although much more accurate than serum screening, does generate a small percentage of null or false results, as explained by the doctor quoted below.

> **Doctor:** *Sometimes, instead of getting the baby's cells growing, what they get is your cells growing, so we get the results back saying 'normal female', but it is you, not the baby. That is very rare, but it sometimes happens. We know it does because they have a boy, when we thought they were going to have a girl. But, as I say, that is very rare. Another rare thing that might happen is that your cells and the baby's cells might get mixed up together, and we might get what we call a mosaic. And then we would not know if it was the baby who had a funny mixture of chromosomes, or if it was your and the baby's chromosomes having got mixed together. Again, those are very rare. Ninety-nine per cent of the time or more you get a straight-forward result without any problems at all.* (Mary, aged 46, hospital consultation [Anderson], 15 weeks, amniocentesis)

Another doctor pointed out that if a mosaic was detected, or other problems invalidated the test, women would be offered a second test, doubling the stated risk of a miscarriage, the price paid for maximal reduction of genetic uncertainty.

> **Doctor:** *The other thing that can sometimes happen is that your cells and the baby's cells can get mixed up together, and we grow what we call a mosaic pattern, so, a mixture of chromosomes . . . And so we would have to offer you a further test, taking a further sample from the baby. Sometimes, the culture doesn't work properly, so you might get word that it has failed, that something has gone wrong with the culture. That happens very rarely these days. But you might be faced with the prospect of having the same test, with the same risk of miscarrying the baby.* (Penny, aged 36 [Lewin], hospital consultation, 12 weeks, amniocentesis)

Waiting for amniocentesis results

Women who proceeded with amniocentesis faced two adverse consequences over and above possible risk of miscarriage: the anxiety caused by waiting up to three weeks for a test result, a delay associated with the length of time taken to culture cells; and the emotional trauma of abortion if an abnormality was detected, and they decided to terminate the pregnancy. The time lag between being tested and receiving the results of amniocentesis was discussed in only three of the 16 hospital consultations. In one, it was mentioned briefly without reference to the anxiety which might ensue.

Doctor: *But then we will let you go home, and we get the results back, usually within two to three weeks after your test. Which will mean that if we are doing the test at about 14 to 16 weeks, which is when we normally do it, you will be 17 or 18 or a bit further on by the time we get the results.* (Charlotte, aged 36 [Fallowfield], hospital consultation, amniocentesis)

Whilst the above doctor did not discuss the significance of this delay, another emphasised that the waiting period could cause considerable distress.

Doctor: *The problem with that amniocentesis is that it's a three-week wait, which is a killer. If you have the blood test today, I'd have you back for the result next week. And then, hopefully, if you did screen positive, and you wanted an amniocentesis that day, you could have it in the afternoon. It's a killer* [waiting for amniocentesis result]. *We get you back in exactly three weeks, but you can't think straight for three weeks. It's dreadful, really . . . You have to take these things into consideration. Also you are bound to have an affected pregnancy.* (Heather, aged 36, hospital consultation [Bell], 16 weeks, no genetic tests)

The quotation raised the possibility that the emotional distress which results from opting for amniocentesis as a risk management strategy might adversely affect the pregnancy, and damage the baby (Mansfield, 1988). As we have noted before in relation to the above consultation, the doctor's willingness to discuss drawbacks so openly may have resulted from awareness of this woman's decisive prior rejection of genetic screening/testing.

Pregnancy termination

If an abnormality was detected, women were faced with the prospect of a late termination, on account of the 3-week waiting period for amniocentesis results. As pointed out in Chapter 5, doctors tended not to dwell on this distressing but unlikely process during hospital consultations. It was discussed in only two of the 16 hospital consultations. Doctors' reticence protected women, nearly all of whom would not be affected, from short-term stress, but deprived them of information relevant to their decision-making. Similarly, Kolker and Burke (1994, p. 54) found that only seven out of 23 genetic counsellors regularly discussed, or offered to discuss, the nature of abortion procedures. Rothman (1988, pp. 38–9) observed a similar reticence about abortion in her study of prenatal genetic counselling in the USA.

The quotation given below at least points to the emotional significance for a woman of undergoing labour after terminating her pregnancy in order to deliver a dead baby.

Doctor: *So you are looking at, if the result shows that the baby has Down's syndrome, of having a termination when you are 19 to 20 weeks' pregnant, which would involve actually being in labour, delivering the baby, rather than going to sleep and waking up and being done with like that. That is something that you need to know about.* (Margaret, aged 35, hospital consultation [Anderson], serum screening)

Although an unlikely contingency for most women, this logical endpoint gave the genetic screening/testing system its main purpose. Women could not make informed choices in ignorance of its meaning.

We may speculate as to why doctors did not reveal the details of termination, given the conscientious, careful explanations of genetic screening/testing which they provided. Doctors may have wanted to avoid alarming women about an improbable contingency. One doctor explained such reticence as follows.

Interviewer: *Do you discuss termination at all when you discuss the screening and amnio?*
Doctor: *Not a lot, no . . . I mean I tend to keep off at that stage. I don't want to go any further.*
Interviewer: *Why?*
Doctor: *I don't know. I just feel that, having to, they come for the booking clinic hoping that everybody will be nice to them, and they will be seeing the baby scan and pictures and all that. I don't want to ruin that. I don't want to talk about the negative side of all of that.* (Minto, interview)

Withholding such information avoided emotional damage arising from reflection on a relatively unlikely contingency, but left women unable to make fully informed decisions about genetic test options. If they decided to be tested, and the results proved positive, they could not then get back to the situation of having no knowledge about their baby's genetic status. The tactics adopted by another doctor suggest an attempt to steer between the two horns of this risk communication dilemma.

> **Doctor:** *I don't go into the gory details of what a mid-trimester termi-nation means, but I would say that it would involve going through a labour.*
> (Bell, doctor, interview)

This communication dilemma will be found whenever health profes-sionals impart probabilistic information about uncommon adverse events. Spelling out such contingencies enables service users to make informed choices, but causes widespread distress about mostly unlikely contingencies.

Conclusions

It is not possible to generalise about the specific properties of the screening system explored in this book. On the contrary, a broad sweep analysis of a single case shows that such systems operate as complex totalities in which the formal, evidence-based specification provides only one component. Other elements include: the translation, more or less, of system design into operational practice; the communication of risk information to service users navigating such systems; the power relationships between practitioner groups; and the wider cultural backdrop of relevant social attitudes. In the UK at least, where access to health services for the majority of the population which uses the NHS is determined by locality, prenatal genetic screening provides a good example of the well-known postcode lottery. The rapid pace of change in genetic screening and other technologies, which local health-care systems respond to at different rates, can only increase local organisational variability.

Although no descriptive generalisations can be drawn from our study, it does suggest some hypotheses about the operation of screening systems designed to prevent uncommon events. These are listed below, together with brief pointers to their implications for practice.

1. Risks are constituted by screening systems (Chapter 1)

The homogeneity and negativity of the risk entities which screening systems are designed to prevent tend to become taken for granted. We found evidence in our case study that doctors mostly presumed parental knowledge of the symptomology of Down's syndrome despite the underlying variability of its manifestation. But service users cannot make informed choices unless the nature, often problematic and constructed, of the risk in question is brought onto the agenda.

2. Risk management is shaped by wider cultural attitudes (Chapters 1 and 2)

Risk judgements are influenced by complex, culturally mediated but personally variable beliefs. Our case study showed that women's attitudes towards genetic screening and testing were influenced by their views about disability, ageing, pregnancy and abortion. Service providers need both to take account of such beliefs and to appreciate their influence on their own clinical judgements.

3. The incorporation of service user choice into system design gives rise to social inequalities (Chapter 3)

Inevitably, the exercise of consumer choice becomes socially patterned. Our study showed that better-off women were more likely to be offered genetic tests because they were more likely to request them. Service providers need to recognise and tackle such inequalities.

4. The behaviour of screening systems does not match their design specification (Chapter 3)

Even apparently simple screening criteria such as age may prove surprisingly difficult to translate into organisational practice. In our study, we found that a significant proportion of higher risk women aged 35 and over were not offered genetic tests, even though they wished to receive them. Such lacunae arose from organisational complexities and pressures, for example the non-recording of maternal age on the case notes which doctors were given. The operation of screening systems according to their specification should not be taken for granted, nor organisational difficulties underestimated.

5. The operation of screening systems is determined by the interaction of population and case-based considerations (Chapter 3)

As noted in the Introduction, tension can be expected between the new nomothetic screening approach, which is oriented towards the processing of populations, and an idiographic case-based orientation which focuses on the concerns of individuals. Our study showed that women who were concerned about the health of their baby were more likely to be offered genetic tests, regardless of the reason. Doctors acknowledged that they might offer genetic tests as a form of reassurance, and that they felt inhibited from delving into women's personal circumstances.

This process entails risk abstraction, with one kind of risk concern managed through a causally unconnected preventative intervention. Screening offers should not be used as a substitute for consideration of other concerns simply because of their availability.

6. The specification of screening systems is influenced by resource constraints (Chapter 3)

The categorisation of individuals as at low risk can be used to legitimate the exclusion of this group from costly screening processes. A substantial proportion of women would have liked to be, but were not, offered genetic tests. Although they belonged, mostly, to the defined lower risk group, this distinction would have shifted if the hospital had offered a universal service, as consultants wished, and as is done in many other maternity centres. The distinction between high and low risk cannot be based on numerical probability alone, and entails a value judgement about what probability level is acceptable in a particular context. Service providers should avoid using this distinction to rationalise resource constraints.

7. Divisions between higher and lower risk groups become reified (Chapter 4)

Organisationally driven divisions of service users into higher and lower risk groups can give rise to the illusion that the borderline between them marks a qualitative distinction. More than one woman who participated in our study described the transition to the higher risk group at the age of 35 as magical, and some expressed scepticism about the medical grounds for this apparent metamorphosis. Institutionalised distinctions between higher and lower risk groups should not be confused with the continuous shifts in risk which they dissect.

8. Risk managers face the dilemma that offering the higher risk group only more intense interventions reduces their take-up rate (Chapter 4)

Risk management systems often contain intervention options of varying intensity, with the stronger ones offering more protection, but causing more side-effects, and therefore deemed more appropriate for higher risk cases. Risk managers face the following dilemma. Offering the higher risk group only the more intense intervention may reduce their uptake of any preventative measure. However, offering them the full range of options may increase the proportion of high risk cases who opt for preventative measures which official opinion deems inadequate. Our case study showed that women offered only amniocentesis were more likely to accept it than those given a choice between amniocentesis and serum screening, but were also more likely to remain untested. Service providers seeking to channel the highest risk group towards the most intense intervention need to recognise this dilemma.

9. Risk communicators must balance the need to avoid distress about unlikely contingencies against the obligation to enable service users to make informed choices (Chapter 5)

Those who operate screening systems need to manage a communication dilemma. On the one hand, spelling out the implications of low probability negative events may potentially distress an entire population even though only a small minority will be affected. On the other hand, not providing this information precludes informed choice. The doctors whom we observed did not usually discuss late termination with pregnant women, on the grounds that they did not wish to alarm them about an unlikely contingency. However, women can not make informed decisions unless they understand the implications of all possible outcomes.

10. Bayesian complexities make the full, neutral communication of probabilistic information problematic (Chapter 6)

The task of informing service users about their probability of an adverse event entails complex Bayesian inductive reasoning which the app-arently simple, scientific nature of numerical statistics conceals. The doctors who participated in our case study often reified rule of thumb use of the probability heuristic, treating probabilities as naturalistic descriptions. However, their communication about probability entailed numerous slants, for example emphasis on the low probability of a false serum screening negative rather than on the much higher chance of a false positive. A more systematic approach to the communication of probabilistic pictures which recognises their complexity is required.

11. Service users are unlikely to be informed about the full decision tree which they are required to navigate (Chapter 7)

Preventative systems can develop considerable structural complexity, making it difficult for service users to grasp their overall structure. In our case study, we found that doctors themselves expressed alarm about the complexity of the decision-tree summarised in Figure 3.1, and rarely described it fully. However, service users, again, cannot make informed choices unless they fully understand the algorithms which they are required to navigate.

12. The operation of risk management systems is predicated on assumptions about the locus of decision-making responsibility (Chapter 7)

As noted in the Introduction, the development of new screening systems offers individuals a greater, although still limited, degree of control over their personal fates, but at the price of having to accept greater responsibility. Contingencies which can be controlled, even probabilistically, must also be managed. Socially mediated assumptions may be made about where such responsibility should fall. Our case study showed that pregnant women were often expected to carry responsibility for genetic decision-making, and sometimes felt unsupported by their partners. Service providers need to avoid gendered or otherwise culturally mediated presumptions about the locus of responsibility for screening decisions.

References

Aarvold, J. (1998) 'Risk, Sex and the Very Young Mother', in B. Heyman (ed.) *Risk, Health and Health Care: a Qualitative Approach*, Edward Arnold.

Aarvold, J. and C. Buswell (1999) 'Young Mothers: Whose problem?', *Youth & Policy*, **64**, 1–14.

Abuelo, D.N., M.R. Hopmann, H.G. Barsel-Bowers and A. Goldstein (1991) 'Anxiety in Women with Low Maternal Serum Alpha-fetoprotein Screening Results', *Prenatal Diagnosis*, **11**, 381–5.

Adams, J. (1995) *Risk*, London: UCL Press.

Advisory Committee on Genetic Testing (2000) *Prenatal Genetic Testing*, London, Health Departments of the United Kingdom.

Ales, K.L., M.L. Druzin and D.L. Santini (1990) 'Impact of Maternal Age on the Outcome of Pregnancy', *Surgery, Gynaecology and Obstetrics*, **171**, 209–16.

Andersen, A.N., J. Wolfart, P. Christens, J. Olsen and M. Melbye (2000) 'Maternal Age and Fetal Loss: Population Based Register Linkage Study', *British Medical Journal*, **320**, 1708–12.

Anonymous (1999) 'Prostate Cancer Screening Tests now Corrected', *Pennsylvania Medicine*, **102**, 10–12.

Armstrong, D., S. Michie and T. Marteau (1998) 'Revealed Identity: a Study of the Process of Genetic Counselling', *Social Science & Medicine*, **47**, 1653–8.

Bailey, R. (1996) 'Prenatal Testing and the Prevention of Impairment: a Woman's Right to Choose?' in J. Morris (ed.) *Encounters with Strangers: Feminism and Disability*, London: The Women's Press.

Beazoglou, T., D. Heffley, J. Kyropoulos, A. Vintzileos and P. Benn (1998) 'Economic Evaluation of Prenatal Screening for Down Syndrome in the U.S.A.', *Prenatal Diagnosis*, **18**, 1241–52.

Beck U. (1992) *Risk Society: towards a New Modernity*, London: Sage.

Beck-Gernsheim E. (1996) 'Life as a Planning Project', in S. Lash, B. Szerszynski and B. Wynne (eds) *Risk, Environment and Modernity: towards a New Ecology*, London: Sage.

Berkowitz, G.S., M.L. Skovron, R.H. Lapinski and R.L. Berkowitz (1990) 'Delayed Childbearing and the Outcome of Pregnancy', *New England Journal of Medicine*, **322**, 659–64.

Bernstein, P.L. (1996) *Against the Gods: the Remarkable Story of Risk*, New York: John Wiley & Sons.

Black, R.B. (1979) 'The Effects of Diagnostic Uncertainty and Available Options on Perceptions of Risk', *Birth Defects: Original Articles Series*, **15**, 341–54.

Blumberg, B.D. (1984) The Emotional Implications of Prenatal Diagnosis, in A.E.H. Emery and M. Pullen (eds), *Psychological Aspects of Genetic Counselling*, London: Academic Press.

Bound, J.P., B.J. Francis and P.W. Harvey (1995) 'Downs-Syndrome: Prevalence and Ionizing-Radiation in an Area of North-West England 1957–91', *Journal of Epidemiology and Community Health*, **49**, 164–70.

Burn, J., S. Fairgrieve, P. Franks, I. White and D. Magnay (1996) 'Audit of Maternal Serum Screening: Strategies to Augment Counselling in Response to Women's Views', *European Journal of Human Genetics*, **4**, 108–12.

Castel, R. (1991) 'From Dangerousness to Risk', in G. Burchell, C. Gordon and P. Miller (eds) *The Foucault Effect*, London: Harvester Wheatsheaf.

Chitty, L.S., G.H. Hunt, J. Moore and M.O. Lobb (1991) 'Effectiveness of Routine Ultrasonography in Detecting Fetal Structural Abnormalities in a Low Risk Population', *British Medical Journal*, **303**, 1165–9.

Collacott, R.A., S.A. Cooper and I.A. Ismail (1994) 'Multiinfarct Dementia in Down's Syndrome', *Journal of Intellectual Disability Research*, **38**, 203–8.

Cooper, S.A. and R.A. Collacott (1994) 'Clinical-Features and Diagnostic-Criteria of Depression in Down's Syndrome', *British Journal of Psychiatry*, **165**, 399–403.

Corbin, J.M. and A. Strauss (1992) 'A Nursing Model for Chronic Illness Management Based upon the Trajectory Framework', in P. Woog (ed.) *The Chronic Illness Trajectory Framework: the Corbin and Strauss Nursing Model*, New York: Springer.

Cuckle, H.S. (1996) 'Established Markers in Second Trimester Serum', *Early Human Development*, **47**, S27–9.

—— (1997) 'Epidemiology of Down Syndrome', in J.G. Grudzinskas and R.H.T. Ward (eds) *Screening for Down's Syndrome in the First Trimester*, London: RCOG Press.

Cuckle, H.S. and N.J. Wald (1990) 'Screening for Down Syndrome', in R.J. Lilford (ed.) *Prenatal Diagnosis and Prognosis*, London: Butterworth.

Cuckle, H.S., N.J. Wald and S.G. Thompson (1987) 'Estimating a Woman's Risk of Having a Pregnancy Associated with Down's Syndrome Using her Age and Serum Alpha-Protein Level', *British Journal of Obstetrics and Gynaecology*, **94**, 387–402.

Davison, C., S. Frankel and G. Davey Smith (1992) 'The Limits of Lifestyle: Reassessing 'Fatalism' in the Popular Culture of Illness Prevention', *Social Science & Medicine*, **6**, 675–85.

Dawson, A.J., M.S. Matharu, M.D. Penney and M. Creasy (1993) 'Serum Screening for Down's Syndrome', *British Journal of Obstetrics and Gynaecology*, **100**, 875–7.

Decker, K.M., M. Harrison and R.B. Tate (1999) 'Satisfaction of Women Attending the Manitoba Breast Screening Program', *Preventive Medicine*, **29**, 22–7.

Delabar, J.M., D. Theophile, Z. Rahmani, Z. Chettouh, J.L. Blouin, M. Prieur, B. Noel and P.M. Sinet (1993) 'Molecular Mapping of Twenty-four Features of Down Syndrome on Chromosome 21', *European Journal of Human Genetics*, **1**, 114–24.

DOH, Welsh Office, Scottish Office, Department of Health and Social Services, Northern Ireland (1998) 'Why Mothers Die: Report of Confidential Enquiries into Maternal Deaths in the United Kingdom 1994–1996', TSO: London.

Donnai, P., N. Charles and R. Harris (1981) 'Attitudes of Patients after "Genetic" Termination of Pregnancy', *British Medical Journal*, **282**, 621–2.

Donnenfeld, A.E. (1995) 'The Risk Figure of 1/270', *Journal of Medical Science*, **2**, 1–2.

Douglas, M. (1990) 'Risk as a Forensic Resource', *Daedalus*, **119**, 1–16.

Douglas, M. (1994) *Risk and Blame: Essays in Cultural Theory*, London: Routledge.

Down Syndrome Abstract (1999) *Down Syndrome Abstract of the Month*, February 1999. http://www.ds-health.com.

Dracup, C. (1995) 'Hypothesis Testing: What It Really Is', *Psychologist*, **8**, 359–62.

Drake, H., M. Reid and T.M. Marteau (1996) 'Attitudes towards Termination for Foetal Abnormality: Comparisons in Three European Countries', *Clinical Genetics*, **49**, 134–40.

Duchon, M.A. and K.L. Muise (1993) 'Pregnancy after Age 35', *The Female Patient*, **18**, 69–72.

Edem, E., B.F. Ekwo, J.K. Seals, R.A. Williamson and J.W. Hanson (1985) 'Factors Influencing Maternal Estimates of Genetic Risk', *American Journal of Medical Genetics*, **20**, 491–504.

Ettore, E. (1999) 'Experts as "Storytellers" in Reproductive Genetics: Exploring Key Issues', *Sociology of Health and Illness*, **21**, 539–59.

Evans, M.I., P.G. Pryde, W.J. Evans and M.P. Johnson (1993) 'The Choices Women Made about Prenatal Diagnosis', *Foetal Diagnosis and Therapy*, **8**, 70–80.

Evers-Kiebooms, G., A. Swerts and H. van den Berghe (1988) 'Psychological Aspects of Amniocentesis: Anxiety Feelings in Three Different Risk Groups', *Clinical Genetics*, **33**, 196–206.

Fairgrieve, S., D. Magnay, I. White and J. Burn (1997) 'Maternal Screening for Down's Syndrome: a Survey of Midwives' Views', *Public Health*, **111**, 383–5.

Falk, R. and C.W. Greenbaum (1995) 'Significance Tests Die Hard: the Amazing Persistence of a Probabilistic Misconception', *Theory & Psychology*, **5**, 75–98.

Featherman, D.L. (1986) 'Biography, Society and History: Individual Development as a Population Process', in A.B. Sorenson (ed.) *Human Development and the Life Course*, Hillsdale, NJ: Erlbaum.

Ferguson-Smith, M.A. (1983) 'Prenatal Chromosomal Analysis and Its Impact on the Birth Incidence of Chromosomal Disorders', *British Medical Bulletin*, **39**, 355–64.

Fischoff, B., S.R. Watson and C. Hope (1984) 'Defining Risk', *Policy Sciences*, **17**, 123–39.

Frets, P.G., H.J. Duivenvoorden, F. Verhage, E. Ketzer and M.F. Niermeijer (1990) 'Model Identifying the Reproductive Decision after Genetic Counseling', *American Journal of Medical Genetics*, **35**, 503–9.

Furlong, R.M. and R.B. Black (1984) 'Pregnancy Termination for Genetic Indications: the Impact on Families', *Social Work in Health Care*, **10**, 17–34.

Gardosi, J., T. Mul, M. Mongelli and D. Fagan (1998) 'Analysis of Birthweights and Gestational Age in Antepartum Stillbirths', *British Journal of Obstetrics and Gynaecology*, **105**, 524–30.

Giddens, A. (1991) *Modernity and Self-Identity: Self and Politics in the Late Modern Age*, Oxford: Polity Press.

Gigerenzer, G., P. Todd and the ABC Research Group (1999) *Simple Heuristics that Make Us Smart*, Oxford: Oxford University Press.

Goel, V., R. Glazier, A. Summers and S. Holzapfel (1998) 'Psychological Outcomes Following Maternal Serum Screening: a Cohort Study', *Canadian Medical Association Journal*, **159**, 651–6.

Greber-Platzer, S., D. Schatzmann-Turhani, G. Wollenek and G. Lubek (1999) 'Evidence against the Current Hypothesis of "Gene Dosage Effects" of Trisomy 21: ets-2, encoded on chromosome 21 is not over expressed in hearts of patients with Down syndrome', *Biochemical and Biophysical Research Communications*, **254**, 395–9.

Green, J.M. (1994) 'Serum Screening for Down's Syndrome: Experiences of Obstetricians in England and Wales', *British Medical Journal*, **309**, 769–72.

Green, J., H. Statham and C. Snowdon (1992) 'Screening for People Abnormalities: Attitudes and Experiences', in T. Chard and M.P.M. Richards (eds) *Obstetrics in the 1990s: Current Controversies*, London: McKeith Press.

Haddow, J.E., G.E. Palomaki, G.J. Knight, J. Williams, A. Pulkkinen, J.A. Canick, D.N. Saller Jr and G.B. Bowers (1992) 'Prenatal Screening for Down Syndrome with Use of Maternal Serum Markers', *New England Journal of Medicine*, **327**, 588–93.

Halliday, J.L, J. Lumley and L. Watson (1995) 'Comparison of Women Who Do and Do not Have Amniocentesis or Chorionic Villus Sampling', *The Lancet*, **345**, 704–9.

Halliday, J.L., F. Lyndsey, J.L. Watson, D.M. Danks and L.J. Sheffield (1995) 'New Estimates of Down Syndrome Risks at Chorionic Villus Sampling, Amniocentesis and Livebirth in Women of Advanced Maternal Age from a Uniquely Defined Population', *Prenatal Diagnosis*, **15**, 455–65.

Hallowell, N. (1999) 'Doing the Right Thing: Genetic Risk and Responsibility', *Sociology of Health & Illness*, **21**, 597–621.

Hansson, S.O. (1993) 'The False Promise of Risk Analysis', *Risk Analysis*, **6**, 16–26.

Harper, P.S. (1991) *Practical Genetic Counselling* (3rd edn), Oxford: Butterworth-Heinemann.

Harré, R. and P.F. Secord (1972) *The Explanation of Social Behaviour*, Oxford: Blackwell.

Heidrich, S.M. and M.S. Cranley (1989) 'Effect of Foetal Movement, Ultrasound Scans, and Amniocentesis on Maternal–Foetal Attachment', *Nursing Research*, **38**, 81–4.

Heyman, B. (1995) (ed.) *Researching User Perspectives on Community Health Care*, London: Chapman & Hall.

Heyman, B. (1998) (ed.) *Risk, Health and Health Care: a Qualitative Approach*, London: Edward Arnold.

Heyman, B. and M. Henriksen (1998a) 'Values and Health Risks', in B. Heyman (ed.) *Risk, Health and Health Care: a Qualitative Approach*, London: Edward Arnold.

Heyman, B. and M. Henriksen (1998b) 'Probability and Health Risks', in B. Heyman (ed.) *Risk, Health and Health Care: a Qualitative Approach*, London: Edward Arnold.

Heyman, B. and S. Huckle (1993) 'Not Worth the Risk? Attitudes of Adults with Learning Difficulties and Their Informal and Formal Carers to the Hazards of Everyday Life', *Social Science & Medicine*, 12, 1557–64.

Heyman, B., M. Henriksen and K. Maughan (1998) 'Probabilities and Health Risks: a Qualitative Approach', *Social Science & Medicine*, **9**, 1295–1306.

Heyman, B., S. Huckle and E.C. Handyside (1998) 'Freedom of the Locality for People with Leaning Difficulties', in B. Heyman (ed.) *Risk, Health and Health Care: a Qualitative Approach*, Edward Arnold.

HMSO (1990) *The Human Embryology Act*, London: HMSO.

Holmes-Seidle, Ryynanen and Lindembaum (1987) 'Parental Decisions Regarding Termination of Pregnancy Following Prenatal Detection of Sex Chromosome Abnormality', *Prenatal Diagnosis*, **7**, 239–44.

Hook, E.B. and G.M. Chambers (1997) 'Estimated Rates of Down's Syndrome in Live Births by One Year Maternal Age Intervals for Mothers Aged 20–49 in a New York State Study: Implications of the risk figures for genetic counselling and cost-benefit analysis of prenatal diagnosis programs', *Birth Defects: Original Articles Series VIII,* **34**, 123–41.

Hook, E.B., D.E. Mutton, R. Ide, E. Alberman and M. Bobrow (1995) 'The Natural History of Down Syndrome Conceptuses Diagnosed Prenatally That Are not Electively Terminated', *American Journal of Human Genetics,* **57**, 875–81.

Horan-Smith, J. and E. Gullone (1998) 'Screening an Australian Community Sample for Risk of Postnatal Depression', *Australian Psychologist,* **33**, 138–42.

Jalbert, P.M. (1996) 'Down's Syndrome Incidence and Paternal Age', *Screening News,* **3**, 5.

Jones, O.W., N.E. Penn, S. Schuchter, C.A. Stafford, T. Richards, C. Kernahan, J. Gutierrez and P. Cherkin (1984) 'Grief Reactions to Perinatal Death: a Follow-up Study', *Prenatal Diagnosis,* **4**, 249–59.

Jongbloet, P.H. and J.H.J. Zwets (1976) 'Preovulatory Overripeness of the Egg in the Human Subject', *International Journal of Gynaecology and Obstetrics,* **14**, 111–16.

Julian-Reynier, C., Y. Aurran, A. Durnaret, A. Maron, F. Chabal, F. Giraud and S. Aymé (1995) 'Attitudes towards Down's Syndrome: Follow-up of a Cohort of 280 Cases', *Journal of Medical Genetics,* **32**, 597–9.

Kolker, A. and M.B. Burke (1994) Prenatal *Testing: a Sociological Perspective,* Westport, CT: Bergin and Garvey.

Lane, K. (1995) 'The Medical Model of the Body as a Site of Risk: a Case Study of Childbirth', in G. Gabe (ed.) *Medicine, Health and Risk: Sociological Approaches,* Oxford: Blackwell.

Laurence, K.M. (1989) 'Sequelae and Support for Termination Carried out for Foetal Malformation', in E.V. van Hall (ed.) *Free Woman: Women's Health in the 1990s,* Lancashire: the Parthenon Publishing Group.

Lawoyin, T.O. (1998) 'Validation and Use of a Simple Device to Identify Low Birth Weight Babies at Birth', *African Journal of Medicine & Medical Sciences,* **27**, 143–5.

Lee, A.J., F.G. Fowkes, G.D. Lowe, J.M. Connor and A. Rumley (1999) 'Fibrinogen, Factor VII and PAI-1 Genotypes and the Risk of Coronary and Peripheral Atherosclerosis: Edinburgh Artery Study', *Thrombosis & Haemostasis,* 81, 553–60.

Lefcourt, H.M. (1992) 'Durability and Impact of the Locus of Control Construct', *Psychological Bulletin* 112: 411–14.

Lehner, P.E. (1996) 'An Introduction to Issues in Higher Order Uncertainty', *IEEE Transactions on Systems, Man and Cybernetics – Part A: Systems and Humans,* **26**, 289–310.

Lehner, P.E., K.B. Laskey and D. Dubois (1996) 'An Introduction to Issues in Higher Order Uncertainty', *IEE Transactions in Systems, Man and Cybernetics – Part A: Systems and Humans,* **26**, 289–92.

Lenaghan, J. (1998) *Brave New NHS? The Impact of the New Genetics on the Health Service,* London: Institute for Public Policy Research.

Lippman, A. (1994) 'Prenatal Genetic Testing and Screening', in A. Clarke (ed.) *Genetic Counselling: Practice and Principles,* London: Routledge.

Lippman, A. (1999) 'Embodied Knowledge and Making Sense of Prenatal Diagnosis', *Journal of Genetic Counselling*, **8**, 224–74.

Lippman-Hand, A. and F.C. Fraser (1979a) 'Genetic Counselling: Provision and Reception of Information', *American Journal of Medical Genetics*, **3**, 113–27.

Lippman-Hand, A. and F.C. Fraser (1979b) 'Genetic Counselling – the Post-counselling Period. I. Parents' Perceptions of Uncertainty', *American Journal of Medical Genetics*, **4**, 51–71.

Lupton, D. (1999) *Risk*, London: Routledge.

Macintosh, M.C.M. (1997) 'What Risks Should Be Given', in J.G. Grudzinskas and R.H.T. Ward (eds) *Screening for Down's Syndrome in the First Trimester*, London: RCOG Press.

Magyari, P.A., B.A. Wedehase, R.D. Ifft and N.P. Callanan (1987) 'A Supportive Intervention Protocol for Couples Terminating a Pregnancy for Genetic Reasons', *Birth Defects: Original Article Series*, **23**, 75–83.

Malm, H.M. (1999) 'Medical Screening and the Value of Early Detection. When Unwarranted Faith Leads to Unethical Recommendations', *Hastings Centre Report*, **29**, 26–37.

Mansfield, P.K. (1988) 'Midlife Childbearing: Strategies for Informed Decision Making', *Psychology of Women Quarterly*, **12**, 445–60.

Marino, B. (1993) 'Congenital Heart-Disease in Patients with Down's Syndrome: Anatomic and Genetic Aspects', *Biomedicine & Pharmacotherapy*, **47**, 197–200.

Marriott S., J. Pelz and J. Kunze (1990) 'Why do Women not Utilise Prenatal Diagnosis?', *Journal of Psychosomatic Obstetrics and Gynaecology*, **11**, 41–51.

Marteau, T.M. (1995) 'Towards Informed Decisions about Prenatal Testing: a Review', *Prenatal Diagnosis*, **15**, 1215–26.

Marteau, T.M., J. Kidd, R. Cook, S. Michie, M. Johnston, J. Slack and R.W. Shaw (1991) 'Perceived Risk not Actual Risk Predicts Uptake of Amniocentesis', *British Journal of Obstetrics and Gynaecology*, **98**, 282–6.

Marteau, T.M., R. Cook, J. Kidd, S. Michie, M. Johnston, J. Slack and R.W. Shaw (1992a) 'The Psychological Effects of False-Positive Results in Prenatal Screening for Foetal Abnormality: a Prospective Study', *Prenatal Diagnosis*, **12**, 205–14.

Marteau, T.M., J. Kidd, R. Cook, S. Michie, M. Johnston, J. Slack and R.W. Shaw (1992b) 'Psychological Effects of Having Amniocentesis: Are These Due to the Procedure, the Risk or the Behaviour?', *Journal of Psychosomatic Research*, **36**, 395–402.

Marteau, T.M., M. Plenicar and J. Kidd (1993) 'Obstetricians Presenting Amniocentesis to Pregnant Women: Practice Observed', *Journal of Reproductive and Infant Psychology*, **11**, 3–10.

Marteau, T.M. and M. Richards (1996) *The Troubled Helix: Social and Psychological Implications of the New Human Genetics*, Cambridge: Cambridge University Press.

Marteau, T.M., J. Slack, J. Kidd and R.W. Shaw (1992) 'Presenting a Routine Screening Test in Antenatal Care: Practice Observed', *Public Health*, **106**, 131–41.

Martin, C. (1992) 'How Do You Count Maternal Satisfaction? A User-Commissioned Survey of Maternity Services', in R.H. Roberts (ed.) *Women's Health Matters*, London: Routledge.

McGrother, C.W. and B. Marshall (1990) 'Recent Trends in Incidence, Morbidity and Survival in Down's Syndrome', *Journal of Mental Deficiency Research*, **34**, 49–57.

McKinlay, J.B. (1982) 'From "Promising Report" to "Standard Procedure": Seven Stages in the Career of a Medical Innovation', in J.B. Milbank (ed.) *Technology and the Future of Health Care, Milbank Reader*, vol. 8. Cambridge, MA: MIT Press.

Meaney, J.F., S.M. Riggle and G.C. Cunningham (1993) 'Providers and Consumers of Prenatal Genetic Services: What Do the Data Tell Us?', *Foetal Diagnosis and Therapy*, **8** (Suppl. 1), 18–27.

Meyer, C., J. Witte, A. Hildmann, K.H. Hennecke, K.U. Schunck, K. Maul, U. Franke, H. Fahnenstich, H. Rabe, R. Rossi, S. Hartmann and L. Gortner (1999) 'Neonatal Screening for Hearing Disorders in Infants at Risk: Incidence, Risk Factors, and Follow-up', *Pediatrics*, **104**, 900–4.

Meyer, J.W. (1986) 'The Self and the Life Course: Institutionalisation and Its Effects', in A.B. Sorenson, F.E. Weinert and L.R. Sherrod (eds) *Human Development and the Life Course: Multidisciplinary Perspectives*, Hillsdale, NJ: Laurence Erlbaum Associates.

Michie, S. and T. Marteau (1996) 'Genetic Counselling', in T. Marteau and M. Richards (eds) *The Troubled Helix: Social and Psychological Implications of the New Human Genetics*, Cambridge: Cambridge University Press.

Mikkelsen, M., A. Hallberg, H. Poulsen, M. Frantzen, J. Hansen and M.B. Peterson (1995) 'The Epidemiologic Study of Down's Syndrome in Denmark, Including Family Studies of Chromosomes and DNA Markers', *Developmental Brain Dysfunction*, **8**, 4–12.

Mili, F., C.F. Lynch, M.J. Khoury, W.D. Flanders and L.D. Edmonds (1993) 'Risk of Childhood-Cancer for Infants with Birth-Defects 2. A Record-linkage Study, Iowa, 989', *American Journal of Epidemiology*, 1993, **137**, 639–44.

Mole, R. (1986) 'Possible Hazards of Imaging and Doppler Ultrasound in Obstetrics', *Birth*, **13**, 29–37.

MRC Working Party on Amniocentesis (1977) 'An Assessment of the Hazards of Amniocentesis', *British Journal of Obstetrics and Gynaecology*, **85**: Supplement 2, 1–41.

Mutton, G., R.G. Ide and E.D. Alberman (1998) 'Trends in Prenatal Screening and Diagnosis of Down's Syndrome: England and Wales, 1989–1997', *British Medical Journal*, **317**, 922–3.

Nelkin, D. and S. Lindee (1995) *The DNA Mystique: the Gene as a Cultural Icon*, New York: Freeman and Co.

Nelkin, D. and M.S. Lindee (1998) 'Cloning in the Popular Imagination', *Cambridge Quarterly of Healthcare Ethics*, **7**, 145–9.

Nelkin, D. and L. Tancredi (1989) *Dangerous Diagnostics: the Social Power of Biological Information*, New York: Basic Books.

Nespoli, L., G.R. Burgio, A.G. Ugazio and R. Maccario (1993) 'Immunological Features of Down's Syndrome – a Review', *Journal of Intellectual Disability Research*, **37**, 543–51.

Neugarten, B.L. (1979) 'Time, Age and the Life Cycle', *American Journal of Psychiatry*, **136**, 887–94.

—— (1996) *The Meanings of Age: Selected Papers of Bernice L. Neugarten*, Chicago: The University of Chicago Press.

Neugarten, B.L. and D.A. Neugarten (1987) 'The Changing Meaning of Age', *Psychology Today*, **21**, 29–33.

Neugarten, B.L., J.W. Moore and J.C. Lowe (1965) 'Age Norms, Age Constraints and Adult Socialization', *American Journal of Sociology*, **70**, 710–17.

Noble, J. (1998) 'Natural History of Down's Syndrome: a Brief Review for Those Involved in Antenatal Screenings', *Journal of Medical Screening*, **5**, 172–7.

Northern Genetics Service (1998) *Maternal Serum Screening in the North of England, 1997*, Newcastle upon Tyne: Northern Genetics Service.

Northern Region Genetics Service (1995a) *Maternal Serum Screening in the Northern Region*, Newcastle upon Tyne: Northern Genetics Service.

Northern Region Genetics Service (1995b) *Maternal Serum Screening in the Northern Region: Information for Health Care Professionals*, Newcastle upon Tyne: Northern Genetics Service.

Oliver, M. (1990) *The Politics of Disablement*, London: Macmillan.

Onolehemhen, D.O. and C.C. Ekwempu (1999) 'An Investigation of Sociomedical Risk Factors Associated with Vaginal Fistula in Northern Nigeria', *Women & Health*, **28**, 103–16.

Petersen, A. (1999) 'Counselling the Genetically "at Risk": the Poetics and Politics of Non-Directiveness', *Health, Risk & Society*, **1**, 253–66.

Phipps, S. and A.B. Zinn (1986) 'Psychological Response to Amniocentesis: 1. Mood State and Adaptation to Pregnancy', *American Journal of Medical Genetics*, **25**, 131–42.

Points, T.C. (1957) 'The Elderly Primipara', *Obstetrics and Gynaecology*, **9**, 348–54.

Prasher, V.P. (1995) 'Overweight and Obesity amongst Down's Syndrome Adults', *Journal of Intellectual Disability Research*, **39**, 437–41.

Press, N.A. and C.H. Browner (1994) 'Collective Silences, Collective Fiction: How Prenatal Diagnostic Testing Became Part of Routine Prenatal Care', in K.H. Rothenberg and E.J. Thomson (eds) *Women and Prenatal Testing: Facing the Challenges of Genetic Technology*, Columbus: Ohio State University Press.

Press, N. and C.H. Browner (1997) 'Why Women Say Yes to Prenatal Diagnosis', *Social Science & Medicine*, **45**, 979–89.

Pueschel, S.M., J.C. Bernier and J.C. Pezzullo (1991) 'Behavioral Observations in Children with Down's Syndrome', *Journal of Mental Deficiency Research*, **35**, 502–11.

Puri, B.K. and I. Singh (1995) 'Season of Birth in Down's Syndrome', *British Journal of Clinical Practice*, **49**, 129–30.

Rapp, R. (1988) 'Chromosomes and Communication: the Discourse of Genetic Counselling', *Medical Anthropology Quarterly*, **2**, 143–57.

Rapp, R. (1994) 'Women's Responses to Diagnosis', in K.H. Rothenberg and E.J. Thomson (eds) *Women and Prenatal Testing: Facing the Challenges of Genetic Technology*, Columbus: Ohio State University Press.

Rapp, R. (1995) 'Risky Business: Genetic Counselling in a Shifting World', in J. Schneider and R. Rapp (eds) *Articulated Hidden Histories: Exploring the Influence of Eric R. Wolf*, California: Public.

Rapp, R. (1999) *Testing Women, Testing the Foetus*, New York: Routledge.

Reichenbach, H. (1949) *The Theory of Probability*, Berkeley University of California Press.

Robinson, J. (1996) 'Epidemiology: Incidence, Prevalence and Size of the Down's Syndrome Population', in P. Gunn and B. Stratford (eds) *New Approaches to Down Syndrome*, London: Cassell.

Roelofsen, E.E.C., L.I. Kamberbeek, T.J. Tymstra, J.R. Beekhuis and A. Mantingh (1993) 'Women's Opinions on the Offer and Use of Maternal Serum Screening', *Prenatal Diagnosis*, **13**, 741–7.

Rook, K.S., R. Catalano and D. Dooley (1989) 'The Timing of Major Life Events: Effects of Departing from the Social Clock', *American Journal of Community Psychology*, **17**, 233–57.

Rose, G. (1985) 'Sick Individuals and Sick Populations', *International Journal of Epidemiology*, **14**, 32–8.

Rose, K.S.B. (1994) 'A Review of Down's Syndrome Studies and Ionising Radiation', *Journal of the British Nuclear Energy Society*, **33**, 145–51.

Rossi, A.S. (1980) 'Life-span Theories and Women's Lives', *Signs: Journal of Women in Culture and Society*, **61**, 4–32.

Rothenberg, K.H. and E.J. Thomson (1994) *Women and Prenatal Testing: Facing the Challenges of Genetic Technology*, Columbus: Ohio State University Press.

Rothman, B.K. (1988) 'The Decision to Have or not to Have Amniocentesis for Prenatal Diagnosis', in K.L. Michaelson (ed.) *Childbirth in America: Anthropological Perspectives*, MA, USA: Bergin and Harvey.

Rothman, K.B. (1994) 'The Tentative Pregnancy: then and now', in K.H. Rothenberg and E.J. Thomson (eds) *Women and Prenatal Testing: Facing the Challenges of Genetic Technology*, Columbus: Ohio State University Press.

Royal College of Midwives (1966) *Preparation for Parenthood*, London: Royal College of Midwives.

Royal Society (1992) *Risk: Analysis, Perception and Management. Report of a Royal Society Study Group*, London: The Royal Society.

Ruchelli, E., A. Uri, L. Duncan, J. Dimmick, D. Huff and C. Witzleben (1990) 'Severe Infantile Subacute and Chronic Liver-Disease in Down's Syndrome', *Laboratory investigation*, **62**, 7.

Sadler, M. (1997) 'Serum Screening for Down's Syndrome: How much do Health Professionals Know?', *British Journal of Obstetrics and Gynaecology*, **104**, 176–9.

Sagi, M., S. Shiloh and T. Cohen (1992) 'Application of the Health Belief Model in a Study on Parents' Intentions to Utilize Prenatal Diagnosis of Cleft Lip and/or Palate', *American Journal of Medical Genetics*, **44**, 326–33.

Santalahti, P., A.M. Latikka, M. Ryynanen and E. Hemminki (1996) 'Women's Experiences of Prenatal Serum Screening', *Birth*, **23**, 101–7.

Santalahti, P., E. Hemminki, A.R. Aro and H. Helenius (1999) 'Participation in Prenatal Screening Tests and Intentions Concerning Selective Termination in Finnish Maternity Care', *Foetal Diagnosis and Therapy*, **14**, 71–9.

Schloo, B.L., G.F. Vawter and L.M. Reid (1991) 'Down's Syndrome: Patterns of Disturbed Lung Growth', *Human Pathology*, **22**, 919–23.

Schuman, A.N. and T.M. Marteau (1993) 'Obstetricians' and Midwives' Contrasting Perceptions of Pregnancy', *Journal of Reproductive and Infant Psychology*, **11**, 115–18.

Searle, J. (1996) 'Fearing the Worst: Why Do Pregnant Women Feel "at Risk"?', *Australia and New Zealand Journal of Obstetrics and Gynaecology*, **36**, 279–87.

Seth, J. and A.R. Ellis (1994) 'The United Kingdom National External Quality Assessment Scheme for Screening for Down's Syndrome', in J.G. Grudzinskas, T. Chard, M. Chapman and H. Cuckle (eds) *Screening for Down's Syndrome*, Cambridge: Cambridge University Press.

Shafer, G. (1990) 'The Unity of Probability', in G.M. von Furstenberg (ed.), *Acting under Uncertainty: Multidisciplinary Conceptions*, Boston, Kluwer Academic Publications, Boston.

Shapiro, B. (1997) 'Whither Down Syndrome Critical Regions'? *Human Genetics*, **99**, 421–3.

Shiloh, S. (1996) 'Decision-making in the Context of Genetic Risk', in T. Marteau and M. Richards (eds) *The Troubled Helix: Social Psychological Implications of the New Human Genetics*, Cambridge: Cambridge University Press.

Shiloh, S. and M. Sagi (1989) 'Effects of Framing on the Perception of Genetic Recurrence Risks', *American Journal of Medical Genetics*, **33**, 130–35.

Sicherman, N., A.T. Bombard and P. Rappoport (1995) 'Current Maternal Age Recommendations for Prenatal Diagnosis: a Reappraisal Using the Expected Utility Theory', *Foetal Diagnosis and Therapy*, **10**, 157–66.

Siegel, R.M., T.D. Hill, V.A. Henderson, H.M. Ernst and B.W. Boat (1999) 'Screening for Domestic Violence in the Community Pediatric Setting', *Pediatrics*, **104**, 874–7.

Silverman, D. (1987) *Communication and Medical Practice: Social Relations in the Clinic*, London: Sage.

Smelser, N.J. and S. Halpern (1978) 'The Historical Triangulation of Family, Economy, and Education', in J. Demos and S. Boocock (eds) *Turning Points: Historical and Sociological Essays on the Family*, Chicago: University of Chicago Press.

Smith, D.K., R.W. Shaw and T.M. Marteau (1994) 'Informed Consent to Undergo Serum Screening for Down's Syndrome: the Gap between Policy and Practice', *British Medical Journal*, **309**, 776.

Smith, D.K., R.W. Shaw, J. Slack and T.M. Marteau (1995) 'Training Obstetricians and Midwives to Present Screening Tests: Evaluation of Two Brief Interventions', *Prenatal Diagnosis*, **15**, 317–24.

Sorenson, D.L.S. (1995) 'Life Event Timing Synchrony', *Journal of Nursing Scholarship*, **27**, 297–300.

Spencer, K. (1997) 'hCG and its Subunits in First Trimester Down Syndrome Screening', in J.G. Grudzinskas and R.H.T. Ward (eds) *Screening for Down's Syndrome in the First Trimester*, London: RCOG Press.

Spencer, K. and P. Carpenter (1985) 'Screening for Down's Syndrome Using Serum Alpha-protein: a Retrospective Study Indicating Caution', *British Medical Journal*, **290**, 1940–3.

Spencer, K., V. Souter, N. Tul, R. Snijders and K.H. Nicolaides (1999) 'A Screening Program for Trisomy 21 at 10–14 Weeks Using Foetal Nuchal Translucency, Maternal Serum Free β-Human Chorionic Gonadotropin and Pregnancy-Associated Plasma Protein-A', *Ultrasound in Obstetrics and Gynaecology*, **13**, 231–7.

Statham, H. and J. Green (1993) 'Serum Screening for Down's Syndrome: Some Women's Experiences', *British Medical Journal*, **30**, 174–6.

Strauss, A. and J. Corbin (1990) *Basics of Qualitative Research: Grounded Theory Procedures and Techniques*. Newbury Park: Sage.

Sullivan, A. and B. Kirk (1999) *Decision-making Dilemmas in Prenatal Diagnosis*, Paper presented at the Risk and Choice: Is There a Conflict? conference, Swanwick, Derbyshire, 29 November, 1999.

Suppes, P. (1994) 'Qualitative Theory of Subjective Probability', in G. Wright and P. Ayton (eds), *Subjective Probability*, Chichester: John Wiley.

Süskind, P. (1987) *Perfume: the Story of a Murderer*, Harmondsworth: Penguin.
Tabor, A., J. Philip, J. Madesen, J. Bang, E.B. Obel and B. Norgaard-Pendersen
(1986) 'Randomised Controlled Trial of Genetic Amniocentesis in 4606 Low
Risk Women', *Lancet*, **1** (8493), 1287–93.
Tajfel, H. (1982) *Social Identity and Intergroup Relations*, Cambridge: Cambridge
University Press.
Tew, M. (1990) *Safer Childbirth: a Critical History of Maternity Care*, London:
Chapman and Hall.
Tolmie, J.L. (1995) 'Chromosome Disorders', in M.J. Whittle and J.M. Connor
(eds) *Prenatal Diagnosis in Obstetric Practice*, 2nd edn, London: Blackwell
Science.
Tuck, S.M., P.L. Yudkin and A.C. Turnbull (1988) 'Pregnancy Outcome in Elderly
Primigravidae with and without a History of Infertility', *British Journal of
Obstetrics and Gynaecology*, **95**, 230–7.
Tversky, A. and D. Kahneman (1971) 'Belief in the Law of Small Numbers',
Psychological Bulletin, **76**, 105–10.
Tversky, A. and D. Kahneman (1973) 'Availability: a Heuristic for Judging
Frequency and Probability', *Cognitive Psychology*, **5**, 207–32.
Van Riper, M., C. Ryff and K. Pridham (1992) 'Parental and Family Well-being in
Families of Children with Down Syndrome: a Comparative Study', *Research in
Nursing & Health*, **15**, 227–35.
Viscusi, W.K. (1992) *Fatal Tradeoffs: Public and Private Responsibilities for Risk*, New
York: Oxford University Press.
Wald, N.J. and A. Hackshaw (1997) 'Screening Using Risk Estimation', in J.G.
Grudzinskas and R.H.T. Ward (eds) *Screening for Down's Syndrome in the First
Trimester*, London: RCOG Press.
Wald, N.J., W. Huttly, K. Wald and A. Kennard (1996) 'Down's Syndrome
Screening in UK', *Lancet*, **347**, 330.
Wald, N.J., A. Kennard, J.W. Densem, H.S. Cuckle, T. Card and L. Butler (1992)
'Antenatal Maternal Serum Screening for Down Syndrome: Results of a Demon-
stration Project', *British Journal of Medicine*, **305**, 391–4.
Wald, N.J., A. Kennard, A. Hackshaw and A. McGuire (1998) 'Antenatal Screen-
ing for Down's Syndrome', *Health Technology Assessment*, **2**, whole number.
Wald, N.J., H.C. Watt and A.K. Hackshaw (1999) 'Integrated Screening for Down's
Syndrome on the Basis of Tests Performed during the First and Second
Trimesters', *New England Journal of Medicine*, **341**, 461–7.
Wertz, D.C., S.R. Janes, J.M. Rosenfield and R.W. Erbe (1992) 'Attitudes towards
the Prenatal Diagnosis of Cystic Fibrosis: Factors in Decision Making among
Affected Families', *American Journal of Human Genetics*, **50**, 1077–85.
White-van Mourik, M.C.A. (1994) 'Termination of a Second-Trimester Preg-
nancy', in A. Clarke (ed.) *Genetic Counselling: Practice and Principles*, London:
Routledge.
White-van Mourik, M.C.A., J.M. Connor and M.A. Ferguson-Smith (1992) 'The
Psychosocial Sequelae of a Second-Semester Termination of Pregnancy for
Foetal Abnormality', *Prenatal Diagnosis*, **12**, 189–204.
WHO (1980) *International Classification of Impairments, Disabilities and Handicaps:
a Manual of Classification Relating to the Consequences of Disease*, Geneva: WHO.
Willis, E. (1998) 'The "New" Genetics and the Sociology of Medical Technology',
Journal of Sociology, **34**, 170–83.

Wynne, B. (1996) 'May the Sheep Safely Graze? A Reflexive View of the Expert–Lay Knowledge Divide', in S. Lash, B. Szerszynski and B. Wynne (eds) *Risk, Environment and Modernity: towards a New Ecology*, London: Sage.

Zepelin, H., R.A. Sills and M.W. Heath (1987) 'Is Age Becoming Irrelevant: an Exploratory-Study of Perceived Age Norms', *International Journal of Aging & Human Development*, **24**, 241–56.

Ziskin, M.C. (1999) 'Intrauterine Effects of Ultrasound: Human Epidemiology', *Teratology*, **59**, 252–60.

Name Index

Subject Index

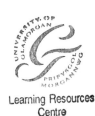